THE COLLEGE WELLNESS GUIDE

1st Edition

Casey Rowley Barneson and
the Staff of The Princeton Review

princetonreview.com

Penguin
Random
House

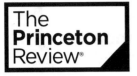

The Princeton Review
110 East 42nd Street, 7th Floor
New York, NY 10017

Published in the United States by Penguin Random
House LLC, New York, and in Canada by Random House
of Canada, a division of Penguin Random House Ltd.,
Toronto.

Terms of Service: The Princeton Review Online Companion
Tools ("Student Tools") for retail books are available for
only the two most recent editions of that book. Student
Tools may be activated only twice per eligible book
purchased for two consecutive 12-month periods, for a
total of 24 months of access. Activation of Student Tools
more than twice per book is in direct violation of these
Terms of Service and may result in discontinuation of
access to Student Tools Services.

ISBN: 978-0-593-45039-0
eBook ISBN: 978-0-593-45038-3
ISSN: 2766-7499

The Princeton Review is not affiliated with Princeton
University.

If there are any important late-breaking developments,
changes, or corrections to the materials in this book, we
will post that information online in the Student Tools.
Register your book and check your Student Tools to see if
there are any updates posted there.

Editors: Aaron Riccio and Anna Goodlett
Production Editors: Emma Parker and
                    Emily Epstein White
Production Artist: Deborah Weber

Printed in the United States of America.

10 9 8 7 6 5 4 3 2 1

1st Edition

Editorial

Rob Franek, Editor-in-Chief
David Soto, Director of Content Development
Stephen Koch, Student Survey Manager
Deborah Weber, Director of Production
Gabriel Berlin, Production Design Manager
Selena Coppock, Director of Editorial
Aaron Riccio, Senior Editor
Meave Shelton, Senior Editor
Christopher Chimera, Editor
Anna Goodlett, Editor
Eleanor Green, Editor
Orion McBean, Editor
Patricia Murphy, Editorial Assistant

Penguin Random House Publishing Team

Tom Russell, VP, Publisher
Alison Stoltzfus, Publishing Director
Brett Wright, Senior Editor
Amanda Yee, Associate Managing Editor
Ellen Reed, Production Manager
Suzanne Lee, Designer
Eugenia Lo, Publishing Assistant

For customer service, please contact **editorialsupport@review.com**,
and be sure to include:

• full title of the book

• ISBN

• page number

Contents

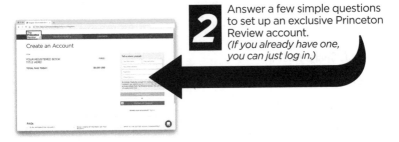
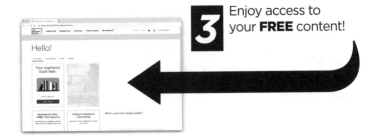

Once you've registered, you can...

- If you're thinking about transferring between colleges, use our searchable rankings of *The Best 387 Colleges* to find more information

- Print additional copies of the activities in this book to help you refine and practice your routines

- Review a compact guide of web resources that can be consulted for additional outreach

- Check to see if there have been any corrections posted for this edition

Need to report a potential **content** issue?

Contact **EditorialSupport@review.com** and include:

- full title of the book
- ISBN
- page number

Need to report a **technical** issue?

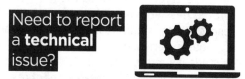

Contact **TPRStudentTech@review.com** and provide:

- your full name
- email address used to register the book
- full book title and ISBN
- Operating system (Mac/PC) and browser (Firefox, Safari, etc.)

Foreword

For over two decades, I've been working here at the glorious The Princeton Review, thrilled to be able to speak at near countless numbers of high schools and colleges campus alike. I count myself among the very lucky to be able to work with students, parents, and counselors near daily, supplying them with need-to-know content about the college process in all its varied parts.

For thirty years, we've been the proud creators of the annual editions of our Best Colleges series, a data- and student-opinion-rich tome with one driving purpose: helping students find their best-fit schools. Adding to the list, in 2003, we started actively surveying high school students and families, speaking directly to their experiences in our (still annual) College Hopes and Worries survey. I remain deeply proud to stand behind titles like *The K&W Guide to Colleges for Students with Learning Differences, Paying for College,* and *College Admissions 101,* which work hand-in-hand to ensure that application, financial, and best-fit concerns are addressed head-on and with confident ease.

For all of these resources, however, I've remained acutely aware of one simple fact: the stress that students feel while searching for, touring, applying, and accepting a school doesn't end when they cross that academic milestone. Higher education is a crucial step in one's career, and we can play a part in making sure that there are no missteps. As we've seen over the last year with COVID-19, especially for students who have had to adjust to being remote, the campus experience plays a monumental role in helping to manage a student's stress, and our full team here at The Princeton Review wanted students to be aware of all those opportunities.

That's where the book you're holding in your hands, *The College Wellness Guide,* comes from. Driven by the expertise and research of my longtime colleague Casey Rowley Barneson, we've broken down the various types of stress the average student may face over their college years into three main categories: mental, physical, and social health. Each chapter looks at different on-campus facilities and resources you can avail yourself of, like finding the right counselor or support setting, or making sure that your body gets the right sort of exercise or nutrition to help the mind stay focused and sharp. And because we know it can be a herculean effort to motivate oneself in a vacuum, we look as well at how helpful it can be to surround yourself with the right friends, whether you're studying or relaxing together. We've even included some stress-relieving tools for your future career and financial health so that you leave college as prepared and excited for the next step as I hope you are right now in readying yourself for your next semester.

Here's a secret that I can share with you that I've learned and learned well from the many students I've spoken with over the years: *you've so got this!* This is what I've uttered, muttered, and much more likely SHOUTED FROM THE ROOFTOPS to students looking to improve their grades or who are worried about the future, and that's because it's the bona fide simple truth. As long as you're willing to put in the work—or in this case, make use of the ample resources on your campus—you can vastly improve your experiences. I'm supremely hopeful that you'll take us up on the tips throughout this book and that you'll give each activity an earnest effort, because at the end of the day, you have the awesome power to succeed wildly!

I'll leave you with one of my favorite quotes from a Mary Oliver poem. "Tell me, what is it you plan to do with your one wild and precious life?" In my mind—you can do anything.

Be well, friends.

Rob Franek
Editor-in-Chief
The Princeton Review

Introduction

The *College Wellness Guide* has been developed from Casey's first-hand experience with students who aren't aware of all the wellness resources available to them in college. She has worked to help countless students gain admission to higher education and find the right strategies and support to meet the rising demands of university life. As students successfully navigate college life and fully embrace their strengths and talents after finding these offerings, they are more apt to succeed in classes, career goals, and managing their daily lives. The tools in this book have been developed to help equip you with:

- the knowledge to advocate for yourself and your needs

- the foresight to stay ahead of mental health challenges

- the opportunity to utilize things that will make you healthier physically, mentally, and socially

- the ability to better manage stress and anxiety

Remember, your development doesn't stop once you are accepted to college. After enrolling, you need to make the most of your time on campus so that you not only graduate but do so with a healthy foundation that will keep you ahead of the curve in your future career. Don't let anything hold you back from your dreams.

In the following pages, you'll take an active role in building a framework that will help to support every key aspect of your overall well-being: physical, mental, and social. You'll learn how to utilize existing services—support programs, campus amenities, learning opportunities, and student communities—and how to find creative and effective ways to satisfy any unmet needs. We'll talk about how to address immediate issues like homesickness, anxiety, depression, and relationship challenges by tracing them to their underlying causes. We'll focus on building or maintaining healthy mindsets that can help you withstand any challenge, even after college. We'll provide strategies to tackle foreseeable challenges including career and financial planning and tips to proactively manage your time and academic course load.

A Wake-Up Call

If you're feeling overwhelmed, know that you're not alone. Above-average levels of stress are commonly cited among students, with 40% of students at one point or another finding their workloads to be hopeless.

Anxiety and depression are among the biggest impediments to academic performance. By reading this book and empowering yourself to make a more supportive environment, you are making sure that you can focus on earning your chosen degree, as opposed to majoring in being stressed.

Options

Identify the things on campus that will empower you. Don't stop at just one thing, like making an appointment with a counselor. Make sure you build a network of alternatives so that if one thing is stressing you out, the rest of your options can help to carry you forward.

Just as you don't go to college for a single class, but rather for a whole well-rounded education, so too can you avail yourself of all the resources of your college. Mental health services, sure, but also facilities to support your physical and social well-being, whether that's healthier food options to keep you fueled, finding classmates and professors who keep you motivated, or making time for restorative walks or meditations between classes so that the words in your textbooks stop blurring.

College should, ideally, let you feel safe and secure enough to try new things and do your best at them. So identify the things you need, the things you want, and keep track of which services are of most use to you. Maybe there's a program tailored specifically to your background or career track, or a class that helps with organization, time management, and study strategies. Maybe there's a service that can safely get you home from a massive party, should you feel uncomfortable.

Notice the type of classroom or campus environment that leads you to participate or stand out. If you're at a big university and a majority of your classes have had a large number of students, how do you find smaller groups to open up opportunities for things like mentorships? If you prefer small discussion-based classrooms, how do you work with an academic advisor to advocate for classes you know you'll feel more comfortable in? What if you have a learning difference but want to work on managing your own schedule rather than asking for support unless absolutely needed? Academics can be stressful, especially when a new semester starts and you are tackling material with which you are unfamiliar.

Opportunities

College is an opportunity for you to create the type of environment where you will thrive. But that's up to you. It doesn't matter how selective the university you're attending is if you feel you can't handle the work, disconnect from classes and friends, and stop leaving your dorm room.

"It will all work out as it's supposed to work out! Or more accurately, maybe, there's no one way things are 'supposed to' work out. Have faith in yourself, in your strength and in your resilience. You will be okay."

—*Tessa, Wellesley*

How to Utilize This Book

Every student's journey is their own. Far be it from us to tell you which chapters to start with, or what you, personally, will find the most useful.

That said, we know that taking the first steps and setting new habits can be difficult, especially when you don't know that you're stuck in a potentially unhealthy routine. To that end, we recommend that you start with the next section, a series of questionnaires, one for each chapter of this book. This will help you identify the areas in which you feel you need the most assistance, and those are the chapters you should start with.

Regardless of which unit (Physical, Mental, Social, or Future Health) and chapter you turn to, you'll find a similarly supportive structure.

Goals

A clear list of goals within the upcoming chapter so that you can identify good habits to develop and trouble spots to avoid.

Visualizations

Visualizations, which appear at the start of each chapter, are brief scenarios that resemble a small sampling of the stories we've heard from other students. We've included these as a reminder of just how common—and surmountable—many stressful situations can be.

Services

Though availability may differ across schools, we strive to highlight the major services you can likely find on any campus, and provides tips and strategies for best utilizing them and immediately destressing.

College Spotlights

Where relevant, we call out some of the offerings and programs initiated by specific schools, which may inspire you to seek the same services at your own.

Activities

Most major sections in a given chapter conclude with some sort of routine-building activity that you can use to put a school's services—and yourself—to the test. Additional pages of these worksheets can be downloaded (for free) from your online student tools.

Reflections

Each chapter ends with an opportunity for you to evaluate how far you've come thus far and where you still have room for growth. Understanding what is and isn't working for you is a vital part of self-care and ensures that you'll keep moving in a positive direction. After all, change rarely happens overnight!

We congratulate you on taking an active step towards becoming the best version of yourself in college. As you go throughout the chapters and begin prioritizing positive habits and your mental health, don't forget to take a moment to see all that you have accomplished. Because your academics will begin to thrive, you'll feel more confident in yourself and your future goals, and you'll be able to have a team of support whenever you need it. You're going to do great.

Student Assessment

Introduction

One of the more insidious aspects of stress is that you're not always aware of where it's coming from. Sometimes you may not even be aware that you *are* being negatively impacted; you just accept feeling lousy as the new normal, a natural part of being in college.

The assessment in this section is designed to help you pinpoint the areas in which you may need more support or where an action plan will be of use to you. There's a 15-question self-evaluation for each of the sections in this book, and I encourage you to begin by taking each of them, even if you think you're totally fine in that area. Once you've finished filling in your answers, your scores will help you to identify where you may have had blinders on, and you can focus first on the tools and coping mechanisms in those chapters. In many ways, it's like studying for any test; once you know where you need to improve, you can focus on that subject and improve your overall grades. Likewise, once you've assessed your needs, you'll be able to better address specific areas of wellness that are important to you, whether those are mental, physical, or social.

Bear in mind that each semester will challenge you in different ways, and you may want to return to this assessment (I encourage you to do so!) to either see how you've grown or to refocus on an area that's holding you back.

Begin by reading through each question and answering as honestly as you can. There are no "right" answers, so take your time and respond genuinely. Afterward, add up your total points for each category and decide which chapter's resources, tips, and guidance can be of most immediate use to you. Once you've addressed those needs, consider looking back through some of the other chapters, as you can always find additional resources to improve a system that works for you.

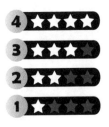

Counseling

Strongly agree = 4	Agree = 3	Neutral = 2	Disagree = 1

_____ **1.** I often try avoiding situations or people that make me anxious.

_____ **2.** I often overplan for every scenario to feel more in control and to reduce anxiety.

_____ **3.** I tend to focus on the worst-case scenario.

_____ **4.** I constantly doubt myself.

_____ **5.** Activities that usually bring me joy don't provide the same feelings anymore.

_____ **6.** I feel really sensitive to failure, criticism, or rejection.

_____ **7.** Academic achievement is more important to me than sleep, friends, or my physical health.

_____ **8.** I feel like my struggles and setbacks are so encompassing that I feel overwhelmed.

_____ **9.** I don't know where to look for help and I feel a bit lost and alone.

_____ **10.** I often feel better when I give voice to my struggles.

_____ **11.** When I have a plan to tackle challenges, I feel much better.

_____ **12.** When I talk to and listen to others, it helps me put my own problems into perspective.

_____ **13.** I still deal with strong feelings from a past event and would like to learn how feel more confident in tackling the day-to-day issues.

_____ **14.** I'd like to find strategies to be able to build consistent, healthy habits and to learn how to incorporate them into my daily routine.

_____ **15.** I benefit from hearing others discuss their problems and then doing workshops based on overcoming them.

Score your self-survey: _____

Support

| Strongly agree = **4** | Agree = **3** | Neutral = **2** | Disagree = **1** |

_____ 1. I found freshman orientation useful in introducing me to resources around campus that I've since used.

_____ 2. Knowing my university prioritizes mental health is important to me.

_____ 3. I like when events are held on campus that promote student engagement and provide a sense of community.

_____ 4. I like the idea of a stressless week leading up to finals.

_____ 5. I would attend a health fair sponsored by the university.

_____ 6. I'd like to listen to a guest speaker on a wellness topic I find important.

_____ 7. I'd like to find upper division classmates who will provide tips and strategies that I can use now.

_____ 8. I'd like to find a support group on campus.

_____ 9. I like when my college does fun things for students like having free snacks around finals and concerts in the quad.

_____ 10. I like designated quiet spaces around campus where I'm able to take a break during a busy day.

_____ 11. I like when my housing area offers counseling support and fun programs that bring me and my peers together.

_____ 12. I like knowing there is a student organization advocating for health and wellness throughout campus.

_____ 13. It's important to me that my campus provides tailored support for specific student populations.

_____ 14. I would like to join a club that helps others with mental health issues.

_____ 15. I want my university to help me manage the anxiety and stress that can surround academics.

Score your self-survey: _____

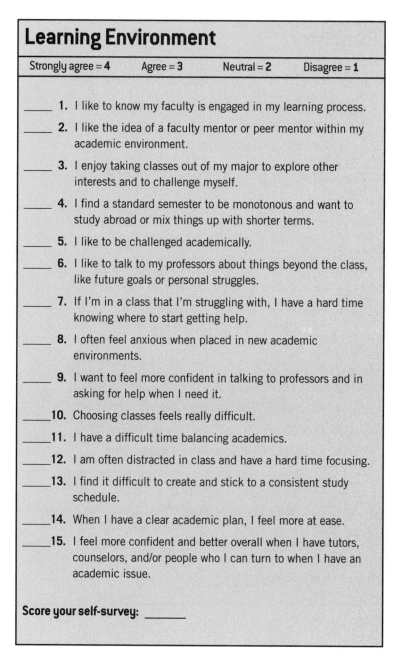

Learning Environment

Strongly agree = 4   Agree = 3   Neutral = 2   Disagree = 1

_____ 1. I like to know my faculty is engaged in my learning process.

_____ 2. I like the idea of a faculty mentor or peer mentor within my academic environment.

_____ 3. I enjoy taking classes out of my major to explore other interests and to challenge myself.

_____ 4. I find a standard semester to be monotonous and want to study abroad or mix things up with shorter terms.

_____ 5. I like to be challenged academically.

_____ 6. I like to talk to my professors about things beyond the class, like future goals or personal struggles.

_____ 7. If I'm in a class that I'm struggling with, I have a hard time knowing where to start getting help.

_____ 8. I often feel anxious when placed in new academic environments.

_____ 9. I want to feel more confident in talking to professors and in asking for help when I need it.

_____ 10. Choosing classes feels really difficult.

_____ 11. I have a difficult time balancing academics.

_____ 12. I am often distracted in class and have a hard time focusing.

_____ 13. I find it difficult to create and stick to a consistent study schedule.

_____ 14. When I have a clear academic plan, I feel more at ease.

_____ 15. I feel more confident and better overall when I have tutors, counselors, and/or people who I can turn to when I have an academic issue.

Score your self-survey: _____

Exercise

Strongly agree = **4**	Agree = **3**	Neutral = **2**	Disagree = **1**

_____ 1. I prefer to exercise in a gym, with structured activities like weightlifting.

_____ 2. I do not have a lot of physical activity in my daily routine.

_____ 3. I am more motivated to exercise outdoors, spreading lots of activity across the whole day.

_____ 4. If my friends joined a workout class with me, I'd be more likely to go.

_____ 5. I want to find a type of workout that I actually enjoy.

_____ 6. I want to have more energy in the day.

_____ 7. I want to find some stress relief from my studies.

_____ 8. Having designated spaces on campus like a recreation center, gym, or track, that I can access anytime for free encourages me to work out.

_____ 9. I don't really see the point in adding exercise into my routine.

_____ 10. I feel a bit intimidated to try a new workout class.

_____ 11. Working out feels like the last thing on my priority list.

_____ 12. I want to exercise, but have no idea where to start.

_____ 13. It's hard for me to stick to a workout routine.

_____ 14. I want to find something non-intensive that gets my body moving, but isn't too much of a commitment.

_____ 15. I am excited about the thought of doing something for myself that would bring me more confidence, joy, and energy to conquer whatever comes my way.

Score your self-survey: _____

Nutrition

Strongly agree = 4	Agree = 3	Neutral = 2	Disagree = 1

_____ 1. No matter how healthily I eat, I feel bad when I indulge my sweet tooth.

_____ 2. I want to find better balance in the foods I eat.

_____ 3. I want to have more energy to be able to make it through a busy day.

_____ 4. It would be helpful to have a better game plan of knowing where to eat so I don't have to overthink when I'm stressed or running late.

_____ 5. I'd like to learn quick meals to help save money by cooking at home.

_____ 6. I often find myself in the library or studying late without access to a dining hall or full meal.

_____ 7. It's important for me to eat healthy, sustainable food.

_____ 8. I want to learn how to cook.

_____ 9. I have a specific diet to maintain and want to know how to better manage my intake.

_____ 10. I feel like I have no idea what eating healthy means.

_____ 11. I like trying local restaurants and new foods, but I also want to save money and not go overboard.

_____ 12. I feel like I have no time to prepare meals or snacks ahead of time.

_____ 13. I'd love to find discounts and food specials for college students.

_____ 14. I'd like to meet with a nutritionist or health professional to better manage my diet.

_____ 15. I don't have any plan when it comes to food, I just eat whatever's available.

Score your self-survey: _____

Study Support

Strongly agree = **4**   Agree = **3**   Neutral = **2**   Disagree = **1**

_____ 1. I need places on campus that are quiet and secluded and where I can study without distraction.

_____ 2. I don't seek out resources like tutoring, study spaces, and office hours.

_____ 3. I struggle with research papers, my grammar, or properly citing sources.

_____ 4. I want to improve my study and time-management skills.

_____ 5. I like when my college organizes campus events that are meant to be fun and stress-relieving for students.

_____ 6. It's important to me that my university has designated study breaks where no classes are held.

_____ 7. Tutoring would help me with specific academic areas.

_____ 8. I want tutoring help, but prefer to find free resources rather than paying for a private tutor.

_____ 9. I work better in study groups.

_____10. I want weekly small-group meet-ups where I can review material I just learned.

_____11. I am in a major that requires preparation for graduate school or more schooling upon graduation.

_____12. It's important to me to know that students are helping advocate for better academics at my university.

_____13. I want to find balance in academics and social activities.

_____14. I have a hard time building a consistent study routine.

_____15. I am often frustrated with my roommate(s) and have a difficult time studying around them.

Score your self-survey: _____

Self-Care

| Strongly agree = **4** | Agree = **3** | Neutral = **2** | Disagree = **1** |

_____ 1. I find it difficult to disconnect when I have a lot of things on my mind.

_____ 2. I tend to stick to the same routine, even when it feels monotonous.

_____ 3. I'd like to break out of my comfort zone and try something new.

_____ 4. I feel overwhelmed with my schedule and often feel like I can't get it all done.

_____ 5. I rarely let myself blow off an assignment even if I'm exhausted.

_____ 6. I find it difficult to focus on one thing, my mind is constantly racing.

_____ 7. I don't usually take time for myself.

_____ 8. I often put others' needs before my own.

_____ 9. Meditation is completely foreign to me.

_____ 10. I'd like to take breaks throughout the day and learn how to refocus but have no idea how.

_____ 11. I am often unorganized with to do lists and find it difficult to decide which tasks to begin first.

_____ 12. I feel like the day just happens to me rather than me taking control of the day.

_____ 13. I tend to consistently hit snooze, finding it difficult to get out of bed right away.

_____ 14. I usually choose studying over sleeping.

_____ 15. Sleep is rarely consistent.

Score your self-survey: _____

Community

| Strongly agree = **4** | Agree = **3** | Neutral = **2** | Disagree = **1** |

_____ 1. I don't feel like I have a core friend group on campus.

_____ 2. I would like to find like-minded peers with similar values and backgrounds that I can relate to.

_____ 3. I have a hard time opening up to new people.

_____ 4. I am often closed off to others and feel safer that way.

_____ 5. I am in a new environment and the thought of making new friends feels intimidating.

_____ 6. I feel like others won't relate to me.

_____ 7. I'd like to find a club on campus to share hobbies and similar interests with peers.

_____ 8. I'd like to join a student organization that holds similar values to those I believe in.

_____ 9. I don't usually take advantage of office hours with professors.

_____ 10. I don't talk to my professors or any faculty outside of class.

_____ 11. It'd be nice to have a faculty member help give me advice on future major and career goals.

_____ 12. It'd be nice to have a peer-mentor provide me with tips and guidance with academics.

_____ 13. I only interact with faculty advisors when I have to pick out classes.

_____ 14. I'd like to join a club, but have no idea where to begin and feel a bit intimidated.

_____ 15. I rarely attend university-sponsored events, even if they seem appealing.

Score your self-survey: _____

Campus

Strongly agree = **4**	Agree = **3**	Neutral = **2**	Disagree = **1**

_____ **1.** I am new to college and have yet to explore campus to the point where I know my favorite spots.

_____ **2.** I'd like to explore the local town, or city more.

_____ **3.** It's important to me to find new experiences and shake up the daily routine.

_____ **4.** I rarely put myself in situations that are out of my comfort zone.

_____ **5.** I feel a bit stuck and would like to find creative ways to find new things to do.

_____ **6.** I have friends, but it'd be nice to have a professional network of students with similar career goals.

_____ **7.** If there was a new exhibit, festival, or fair off-campus, I'd be interested in exploring.

_____ **8.** I'd like to open up internship and prospective job opportunities.

_____ **9.** I'd like to gain new perspectives and learn from others outside of my major.

_____ **10.** I don't feel like I have a core group of people on campus that provide me with guidance and support.

_____ **11.** I'd like to find safe spaces on campus where I never feel judged.

_____ **12.** It's important for me to find like-minded individuals on campus.

_____ **13.** Finding independence in college is important to me.

_____ **14.** Expanding my network in college is important to me.

_____ **15.** Feeling connected and getting to know my community beyond campus is important to me.

Score your self-survey: _____

Career

| Strongly agree = **4** | Agree = **3** | Neutral = **2** | Disagree = **1** |

_____ 1. I am having trouble deciding on and declaring a major.

_____ 2. I don't have a clear idea of my strengths academically.

_____ 3. I have a clear idea of my strengths, but want to have a clear plan on how to apply them to academics and future career planning.

_____ 4. I feel anxious at the thought of making a career decision.

_____ 5. The idea of graduating and getting a job stresses me out.

_____ 6. I am intimidated by resume-writing.

_____ 7. I'd like to create a professional online presence, but have no idea how.

_____ 8. I want to feel more confident in my interview skills.

_____ 9. I have no idea what networking actually means.

_____10. I'd like to feel confident in professional settings.

_____11. I'd like to get an interview, but have no idea where to start.

_____12. I don't know where to find resume-building and career-exploring opportunities.

_____13. I want to find an internship.

_____14. I'd like to talk to successful alumni with similar interests and goals as me.

_____15. It's important to me that I find value in the work I do one day.

Score your self-survey: _____

Finances

Strongly agree = 4	Agree = 3	Neutral = 2	Disagree = 1

_____ **1.** I don't feel like I have a strong handle on my finances.

_____ **2.** When I think about money, I feel anxious.

_____ **3.** I'd like to learn how to save money in college and still have enough left over for fun.

_____ **4.** I want to feel confident in managing my college loans.

_____ **5.** I want to learn tricks that will help me save for my future.

_____ **6.** Feeling secure financially is important to me.

_____ **7.** I would like to know how to manage and pay my own bills.

_____ **8.** I have no idea how to navigate taxes.

_____ **9.** I'd like to create a budget but don't know where to begin.

_____ **10.** I want to find financial freedom.

_____ **11.** No one around me talks openly about money.

_____ **12.** How I was raised as a child has skewed my view of managing money.

_____ **13.** I want to set money aside to travel.

_____ **14.** I want to set money aside for a big goal (like buying a home, a car, etc.).

_____ **15.** Staying on top of finances would help relieve a lot of stress.

Score your self-survey: _____

Scores

Take the scores from each assessment and record them in the table below. Then, turn to the next page and see what to do with each range of scores. You'll note that each of these topics is also the name of a chapter in this book. Once you've used the scores and your personal feelings to determine which areas are your personal priorities, move to the start of that chapter.

Topics	Score
Counseling	
Support	
Learning Environment	
Exercise	
Nutrition	
Self-Care	
Study Support	
Community	
Campus	
Career	
Finances	

Score 40–60

Prioritize the chapters in this range. Scoring above a 40 means you have a strong response to the statements in the survey—these are the areas where you can use the most support. Each of these chapters will not only help you better understand the topic, but also give you advice from current students, professional guidance, and expert tips on how to take control of it.

Score 20–40

Chapters in this range represent areas where you may currently be coping, but likely still have some discomfort. If you have big changes coming up that may impact you—for instance, new classes, or a change in environment—you may want to reinforce these areas by reviewing this chapter, picking up any tools of use to you.

Score 0–20

Congrats! These are the areas where you are the most confident. Read through these chapters to find ways to expand upon your strengths, using the tips and tools to keep growing.

Do What Feels Right For You

The self-assessments you just took are a helpful start toward figuring out what aspects of wellness need a bit more love and attention. While the scores are a helpful indicator of what sections will be most useful, they do not define you and will change over time. These assessments are meant to inform, empower, and inspire you to become a stronger student. This book will help you along the way by providing information and resources to help you:

- Achieve a higher GPA
- Balance academics
- Stand out as a student
- Have more energy
- Have more confidence
- Find purpose in your day-to-day
- Be your biggest advocate
- Take on new challenges

This is your journey, your book, and you have the ability to change the trajectory of your college career. If it helps you to flip around through chapters or activities that catch your eye, go for it. Just be sure to take a moment to pause and reflect, let the advice sink in, take advantage of resources, and remain unafraid to try something new. You just might surprise yourself.

CHAPTER 1

Counseling

In this chapter, we'll discuss how counseling services can be utilized to manage stress caused from academics, the future, and personal experiences. You'll gain insight into various counseling services offered, so you have a clear idea of what to expect and what will work best for you.

You've been dreading an upcoming economics test. You prefer procrastination and usually are able to pull off your work and do well. But this time, it feels different. You're anxious and have been for some time. The stressors this term have been piling up, and it doesn't help that you've had a fight with your roommate. You're trying to manage it all, but you find yourself ditching class and hiding in your room. The anxiety gets so bad that you can barely sleep, you're exhausted, and you miss the economics test entirely.

You've dealt with some mental health issues in the past, but in high school you worked really hard to overcome them and have, for the most part, felt really confident in your coping skills. You're doing well in your classes, and you feel like you're finally able to be yourself with the new friends you've made, but then one week your old feelings creep up and are all too consuming. The confidence you had has completely gone away. You feel like everything you've worked for was for nothing. You see a text from a friend to meet up and you ignore it. What's the point?

Getting into a selective university has been your dream for so long, not to mention a dream for your parents as well. You've been working so hard to attain the grades you feel you can be proud of, and while you've always been able to perform, it seems now that you're here, the pressure of earning good grades and pleasing your family weighs heavily on your shoulders. You begin pulling all-nighters and taking anything that can keep you up through the night and into the early in the morning. But you're noticing you just feel off. Your mood is constantly changing, and you find little purpose in focusing on coursework anymore. You have a few missed calls from your parents, but the thought of calling them back stresses you out. You turn off your phone, shut out your roommate, and hole up in your dorm.

Introduction

Your mental health is important. A study of Boston University enrollees in 2015–2016 found that, at least once a month, over 67% of the students experienced emotional difficulties that affected their academic performance. As you navigate college, counseling support services can help provide you with tools to cope and feel more confident in your ability to tackle whatever comes your way. There are three categories of stressors in college for which you might want to seek mental health counseling: personal, academic, and future. There's nothing that a counselor won't discuss with you, so don't feel like you can't reach out because your problem isn't "severe" enough, or because you're still able to function. Preventing a situation from becoming unmanageable is just as important as helping you feel better. You might face any number of struggles—like depression, homesickness, confusion, trouble studying—throughout your time in college, so it's worth reaching out for help. While turning to a friend for advice might seem less intimidating than heading to the counseling office, your peers might not be equipped to handle everything, despite their best intentions.

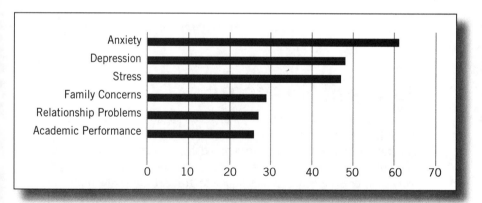

A recent survey of over 500 institutions by the Association for University and College Counseling Center Directors found that anxiety is the biggest concern among students seeking services, followed by depression, family concerns, relationship problems, and academic performance.

Your school believes in you and wants you to succeed—that's why they accepted you—and they're constantly analyzing their services to better support their attendees. Some of the most popular counseling offerings include individual and group therapy, even 24-hour support if you're ever in a crisis.

As your needs change, support services can change with you. While the ways to access services vary between institutions, this chapter will help you figure out where to start. No matter which route you choose, you don't have to go it alone!

Try to take care of yourself. Surround yourself with positive people and stay involved. Get counseling if you need it, define your priorities, and take time for yourself and for friends and families . . . Sometimes you encounter a major issue or have a disability that makes things harder for you. If you know you're one of these people or you figure it out later, it's not the end of the world. There is definitely a solution. Keep your head up and consult the right professionals. There is a way to solve your issue or at least reduce the effects.

—Julian, University of Southern California

Types of Stressors

It is normal for your needs to change throughout college, and to be different from those of your peers. But whether you're a first-generation college student intimidated by a large and unfamiliar campus, a former valedictorian who's overwhelmed by the college workload, or an anxious senior about to graduate in a few months, there's some sort of counseling that can help you. We'll go into more detail regarding the types of counseling available, but it's helpful first to understand things that can impact your mental health.

Personal Stressors

Personal stressors are the things present in your day-to-day life, whether that's grief, loneliness, relationship difficulties, or unhealthy habits. Left unaddressed, they can ripple out to cause anxiety, depression, increased stress, and even suicidal thoughts.

A Counselor Can Help!

Let's say the thought of confrontation cripples you to the point where the stress you're harboring from your roommate who's invaded your space is more than you can stand. A resident advisor or peer-counselor can offer conflict-resolution skills that leave you better equipped to have a diplomatic conversation with your roomie. If you've been struggling with something personally, there are counselors who can help. This is where you *get* to be a little selfish. Personal counseling can help you gain a better understanding of yourself, your strengths, and your future goals.

Breathe and Release

Feeling anxious? Stressed? Try this quick exercise wherever you are to recenter and calm any tense feelings

- Slow your breathing. Breathe in for four counts and breathe out for four counts.

- Squeeze your fists into a tight ball.

- Hold tight for four counts, squeeze and let all the tension ball into your fists.

- Now let go. Notice the tension leaving your fists.

You can tense your shoulders, your arms, any part of your body, and let it go! The nice part is that you can do this wherever you are, without anyone noticing. When you count as you breathe, you begin to quiet any negative thoughts by focusing on counting, and when the tension physically leaves your body, you'll feel lighter. Try it!

Academic Stressors

Let's face it, higher education can knock you off your feet when you least expect it. A lot of that comes with that schedule they hand you at the beginning of each term. If you're a first-year, first-semester student, you may struggle with a schedule that's not as structured as high school. Alternatively, you may face pressure to perform well academically, and the thought of failing one exam or missing a few classes may send you spiraling.

A Counselor Can Help

This is where a counselor can provide you with guidance, accommodations, and solutions to help you manage academic decisions and pressures and hopefully prevent them from negatively impacting your mental health. Over 60% of students who accessed counseling services had a positive impact on their academics, so if you struggle in this area, pick up the phone and schedule a consultation.

Future Stressors

If classes weren't enough, deciding on a career path can really pile on the pressure. Planning your life out feels *really* big. Especially if you're battling finances and feel anxious about your next steps after graduation. Part of growing as an individual is learning how to "adult" in college. While there are a lot of other tools to help you, if you're finding larger life goals weighing heavily on you, counselors can help with that too.

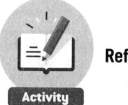

Reframe

Activity

Whatever your future stressors are, you can reframe them. Write down a stressful thought about your future and then rewrite it with a positive spin. Here's an example.

Stressor: It seems like everyone around me has it all together and knows exactly what they want to do.

Reframe: I am excited to allow myself to explore classes and things that interest me, and I know that in time I'll have a clearer idea of what I want to do.

Stressor: _____

_____

Reframe: _____

_____

_____

Stressor: _____

_____

Reframe: _____

_____

_____

Types of Counseling

The type of need you have, and how pressing it is, determines what sort of counseling you'll benefit the most from—and again, this may change throughout your time at school. For example, if you're preparing to take a notoriously difficult class, feel worried about making friends while you study abroad, or are wondering how you'll make rent, your long-term goal could be to develop grounding stress management exercises and strategies with an individual counselor or join group counseling for students with academic anxieties. Alternatively, if you find yourself or a friend in the middle of a mental health crisis, you would need to seek immediate care and reach out to a 24/7 hotline or online service. As you can see, counseling sessions come in many forms for many needs. Don't be afraid to try different forms to find your best fit.

You are not alone and everyone goes through this. Everyone deals with their mental health differently, so be open to looking for a support system that works best for you to improve your mental health.

—Rachel, University of California, Davis

Individual Counseling

Individual counseling or therapy allows you to meet one-on-one with a counselor and discuss a wide variety of issues in a safe, nonjudgmental place. Its goal is to discover ways to cope with and resolve problems you're troubled by. Counselors can help you identify the root of bigger issues, and give you practical tools, help you create goals, and refer you to more guidance in a specific area of need. Best of all, they are an unbiased, open listener. Individual sessions vary in length. Walk-ins or one-off counseling sessions can offer immediate support, while long-term, consistent therapy is an option for those who seek it.

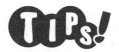

Counseling

If you've never been to counseling, here's what you should know before heading into your first session.

1. Counseling is confidential, mostly. But a counselor's primary role is to make sure you're safe and that includes sharing information with others if you have threatened to hurt yourself or others, or revealed that someone else is endangering you.

2. There's no need to be intimidated by the intake form: whether it's a series of boxes to check or space to fill out, it's just looking to help you explain why you've come so that the counselor can better help.

3. Your first session can be mostly gathering information and gaining insight into your concern. Depending on the counselor, you might also walk away with activities to incorporate into your daily routine.

4. A big part of the counselor's role is to listen. If you feel uncomfortable talking, your counselor may be able to provide additional support. You may also want to consider group counseling.

5. Never feel embarrassed about going to counseling. If it helps, think of it like going to see a tutor for help with classwork, except that the work in this case is non-academic.

Accessing Individual Counseling

Counseling services are embedded throughout campus and finding on-on-one counseling doesn't have to only be with a traditional therapist. Counseling can be housed in a general center on campus with a therapist or counselor, but also in smaller, more specific settings, as with a peer-counselor in your academic department or a residential advisor in your dorm.

There are a few different ways individual sessions can be held to best match your preferences and availability. You can choose from in-person, video chats, or over the phone (both via text or on a call!). There are also variations with frequency and timing. Whether you prefer prescheduled, recurring sessions that are long- or short-term or a one-off drop-in session, there's something available for everyone!

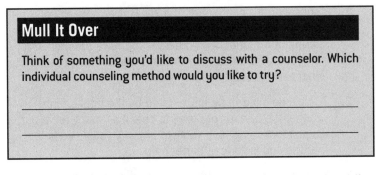

Mull It Over

Think of something you'd like to discuss with a counselor. Which individual counseling method would you like to try?

You will want to research the process of setting up counseling appointments and note when drop-in and regular hours are. There can be waiting times and a delay between the times you request individual counseling and when it is available, so be proactive and reach out early if you think you might want to take advantage of these services.

A majority of schools will offer a few brief therapy sessions for free (or as a part of your fees) and if you need more, will help you navigate next steps. Sometimes your counselor might be able to refer you to a local professional offering discounted or even *pro bono* work. It never hurts to ask!

Group Counseling

Group counseling is another form of counseling where you meet with other people, typically on a regular basis, to discuss similar circumstances or issues, exchange stories and explore solutions with a counselor who will help lead the group and set boundaries. Group counseling can last for a few weeks or longer; it completely depends on the program's structure and the nature of the topic. One of the best things about group counseling is that you are not alone. Groups can be in practically anything too! You can join a group to establish healthy study habits, cope with grief or financial troubles, work through body issues, build resilience, and navigate sobriety.

When looking for a group to join, you should do research on their mission, affiliations, and topics they cover. You can learn a lot about a group by its name and self-description. Here are some examples:

- **Working Together:** Relationships can be complicated. We look at how to effectively communicate with your partner, friend, or family member; understand conflict; and find healthy ways to work together.

- **Managing Anxiety:** Anxiety can be one of the top concerns among college students. Learn how to not only manage your anxiety, but thrive and use tools to remain calm in high pressure environments. Test-anxiety? We cover that too!

- **Family Healing:** Students who have experienced distress from family situations (divorce, substance abuse, unstable home life, financial loss, etc.) are welcome to join this group. We will explore self-worth, personal goal setting, and explore the impact of family experiences.

- **LGBTQ+ Support and Community:** Join our confidential group to find a safe space for emotional support around gender and sexuality. Topics explored will include relationships, self-awareness, and building community.

What to Expect

Group therapy can be beneficial if you're a student wanting to connect with others of similar backgrounds. If you're a first-generation college student, it might be really nice to hear other students share similar struggles and gain some tips from others, especially if you have limited support at home.

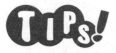

Here are some things to know before your first group session.

- A group leader will set the tone for a safe, confidential space. Your counselor or group leader will ask all members to respect each other's stories and keep whatever is shared in the group.

- There are often icebreakers or exercises that allow you and other members to open up a bit more before diving into a discussion.

- Expect to be challenged, as well as supported. One of the benefits of group counseling is that you hear other perspectives on a similar topic which allows you to explore different outlooks and exchange ideas. It's okay to be a little uncomfortable; that's where the growth happens!

- Plan to show up every week if you can. Most groups meet once a week, and you'll get out of it what you put into it. Mark your calendar and commit to attending.

- Group counseling can be as effective as individual counseling. If it's hard to get an appointment with a counselor individually, try searching for a group that fits.

What's Your Weather Today?

Counselors in group or individual therapy often complete a "check-in" activity or question with their clients to better understand how they're feeling that particular day. Give it a try! Based on how you're feeling today, or this week in general, what is your weather like? Get specific! If you've been having a horrible week, you might be a tornado mixed with hail, or if you're feeling a bit checked out, you might be a sunny day with darker clouds passing in and out. Write out your weather below for how you're feeling:

_____

_____

_____

_____

Access to Group Counseling

Groups can be found typically online with a list of topics, description of what to expect and a schedule. They are often broken up into categories like student success, career, wellness, or mental health. If you can't find a current schedule online, note the contact email or phone number of the organizer and request an up-to-date list. When you follow up, ask about the referral process and see if you need a counselor's referral to join a group, or if you can simply show up. Additionally, check to see if a phone consultation, drop-in or peer counselor is available to share more details about the program. Just as with individual counseling, group sessions can be completed remotely or in-person.

On-Demand Counseling

If you find yourself on a waiting list for a few weeks before meeting with a counselor, some temporary apps and resources can offer some temporary relief. You can talk to non-school affiliated therapists from the comfort of your dorm or apartment, download mindfulness practices, or take guided courses that help you with anything from goal-setting and identifying strengths, to managing anxiety. Other resources include mood surveys and journals or charts that can help you monitor times of the semester where you might be more prone to feeling off. This is also a good way to ease yourself into counseling if you're nervous.

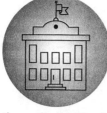

COLLEGE SPOTLIGHT

In response to the rising need of mental-health services, Johns Hopkins University adopted TimelyMD as an online telehealth program free and available to all students. The service includes TalkNow, an online resource staffed by mental health professionals, ready to discuss any issue at any time, the ability to schedule online counseling, and referrals to counseling services at Johns Hopkins, linked with online support. In the initial rollout, over 20% of students were able to access services when traditional counseling offices would otherwise be closed.

Online Programs

It's worth investigating what your university offers regarding online counseling programs. They may have an app that you can download on your phone. One popular resource across campuses is Therapy Assistance Online (TAO Connect). This online program is used by over 150 colleges and universities and is one example of a platform where students can access mental health, substance abuse, and wellness information. Once students log on, they can take self-screenings, and get tips on what modules to work through based on their responses. Do some research and ask your counseling center what online programs like TAO Connect are available to you.

It's great that universities are able to provide the different counseling services, but it is ultimately up to you to be proactive in caring for your mental health. Remember, there's no shame in seeking help, and you should be proud of yourself for taking this big step!

Your mental health is more important than any grade; no school project or class is worth throwing your mental stability down the drain. If your mental health and overall health is taken care of, your ability to perform as a student will be much better. Health comes first; grades and academics follow.

—Chloe, Irvine Valley Community College

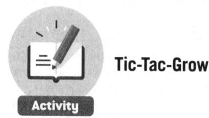

Tic-Tac-Grow

Activity

Knowing what relaxes you can be a great help when speaking with a counselor. When you next feel overwhelmed, pick a new activity from one of the nine categories below. Circle or cross it out, depending on the result. Aim for three circled items in a row, so you have a variety of tools to choose between.

Move Your Body	Socialize	Get Creative
1. Dance around your room	1. Meet up with a friend	1. Journal
2. Take a walk	2. Go to a school event	2. Draw or paint
3. Go for a run	3. Call a relative or long-distance friend	3. Make music
Relax	**Personal Time**	**Nurture Your Mind**
1. Read a book or listen to a podcast	1. Turn off social media	1. Meditate
2. Watch a movie or tv show	2. Order or make your favorite meal	2. Do breathing exercises
3. Take a break to recharge during a busy day	3. Partake in your favorite solo activity	3. Set your intention for the day or week
Nourish Your Body	**Get Organized**	**Serve Others**
1. Hydrate	1. Tidy up your room	1. Volunteer in your community
2. Eat intuitively	2. Organize your inbox	2. Perform a random act of kindness
3. Get a good night's rest	3. Fill in your planner for the week	3. Make a donation

A Note on Suicide Prevention & Emergency Counseling

Suicide is the second leading cause of death among college students. When hearing the word suicide, it might feel uncomfortable or a taboo topic to avoid in any discussion. The reality is, the more we talk about it, the more comfortable we get, which allows more people to access help. Suicidal ideation, thoughts or ideas about dying by suicide, can be caused by depression or drug misuse as well as other factors including social difficulties, stress, academic pressure, performance pressure, poor social relationships, lack of family support, physical or sexual abuse, substance and alcohol misuse, health issues, and bullying. Suicide is preventable.

How to Address Suicidal Thoughts

It can be scary and lonely to experience suicidal ideation and sometimes you may be afraid to tell someone for fear they will "overreact" or that your pain still won't go away. The reality is sharing with a mental health professional, trusted friend, or adult is often the first step in getting the help you need to start feeling better. You have the power. Here are some fundamental things you should know regarding suicide:

1. Know the warning signs. Warning signs can include:

   - Risk factors such as mental health concerns.

   - Previous history with suicide attempts.

   - Dramatic change in behavior.

   - Withdrawing from activities, isolation, irritability, loss of interest in activities.

   - Thoughts or talk about killing yourself or plans to kill yourself, feelings of hopelessness, being a burden to others, feeling trapped.

2. If you notice yourself feeling suicidal, reach out to a trusted friend or adult. Express what you're up against, and that you need their help. They can assist you in obtaining professional support, like a counselor, that you need, while being there for you the best they can.

3. For immediate support, visit contact the National Suicide Prevention Hotline at 1-800-273-8255.

4. If a friend comes to you with suicidal plans or thoughts, do not promise that you won't tell a trusted adult. You have to tell someone to get help for your friend.

Sixty-seven percent of young adults will tell a friend if they are feeling suicidal before telling anyone else.

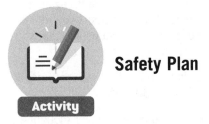

Safety Plan

Work with a trusted adult or professional to come up with a safety plan to activate in case you find yourself in a situation that triggers thoughts and feelings that might lead to suicidal urges. Fill out the following prompts to help you. At the end, write and recite a commitment to executing this safety plan, if it's needed, to a trusted adult, friend, or professional.

My Warning Signs and Triggers

_____

_____

Methods to Calm and Comfort Myself

_____

_____

_____

_____

How to Secure My Environment

_____

_____

My Reasons to Live

1. _____

2. _____

3. _____

4. _____

5. _____

Who to Call

_____
(Name)   (Phone Number)

_____
(Name)   (Phone Number)

_____
(Name)   (Phone Number)

Professional and Emergency Contacts

_____
(Name)   (Phone Number)

_____
(Name)   (Phone Number)

_____
(Name)   (Phone Number)

My Safety Commitment

_____

_____

_____

_____

_____

_____

REFLECTION

What are some struggles that are negatively affecting you personally, academically, and/or future/career wise? How do you feel about your ability to handle them?

_____

_____

_____

_____

Which counseling service sounds most appealing to you and what step can you take right now to access that support?

_____

_____

_____

_____

Look up and register for a suicide prevention training at your college. Write down the most impactful thing you learned.

_____

_____

_____

_____

CHAPTER 2

Support

This chapter gives you a glimpse into nonprofessional mental health resources and organizations on campus that will help you in regard to mental health. You'll hear about campus-wide programming that's built-in to draw attention to and normalize common mental health topics, while simultaneously bringing you relief in your day-to-day. It'll cover different types of student-led organizations that can connect you to peer support, as well as national organizations that are packed with tips and guidance 24/7. Activities along the way will help you note which resources you prefer, as well as challenge you to reach out and access them.

As an introvert, the idea of meeting new people in social settings, or even joining a group study session, causes some anxiety. You're really missing people back home and have been feeling more disconnected than ever before, to the point where you've even considered transferring. You've poured yourself into your studies and not much else, and you rarely leave your room. Homesickness mixed with social anxiety is really starting to take over, but you really want to stick it out and make this place your home.

You just got back to campus from a long summer break and, while you're excited to see your friends, you're a bit apprehensive about this semester. You lost a close family member late last year, and while you've taken time to be home with family and friends. Now that you're back, it feels strange to jump back into university life. Some days you're angry, other days it feels almost normal, and then there are times you just feel tired for no reason at all. You feel like your friends won't really understand and besides, you're over hearing "I'm so sorry, they're in a better place now."

You've dealt with some mental health concerns back in high school that you were able to manage with the help of a counselor and your amazingly supportive brother who's always encouraged you. You began college feeling confident in the coping tools you learned at home, but now that you're here, you feel a bit alienated and sometimes triggered. It's a completely new campus and you feel a bit alone, especially now that your brother is miles away.

Introduction

Most colleges provide students with an online orientation program that identifies the various support services offered on campus. Much of that information includes useful suggestions on how to make healthy choices around drugs, alcohol, and sex; ways to manage stress; and outreach about suicide prevention. But those who don't immediately use these services often forget about them and when they do need help, they're too bogged down in coursework and extracurriculars to know where to go.

You wouldn't build a bridge or a building without any support, so why try to build yourself up throughout college without at least *trying* some of the services offered? There are three main resources that offer programming to support and enhance your mental health: those provided by the school, those generated by student-led organizations, and those available through national organizations.

Campus-wide programming to support your mental health can be embedded into the curriculum, like your freshman orientation, or designated breaks and events in the academic calendar. You may stumble across these by accident, walking by a row of tables where you can sign up for a workshop designed to help cope with depression, or you might find them scheduled for you, like the way some schools integrate a class-free week into the semester so as to reduce the amount of stress on students leading up to finals. These are programs the campus administration has prioritized just for your benefit. Remember, they want you to not only attend the university, but to stay and do well.

Student-led organizations provide platforms to address wellness and are a big part in planning events and spreading mental health awareness throughout campus. Students, after all, are on the ground experiencing college first-hand, and are some of the strongest voices in advocating for positive campus climates. Student organizations and clubs can benefit you in a few ways. For starters, you can find peers struggling or coping with similar mental health issues and extend your community. You can also get involved and be an advocate for changing on-campus policies so as to raise mental health awareness.

Lastly, national organizations like the National Alliance on Mental Illness have the ability to connect you with larger networks, services, and support beyond what's on campus. If you can't find what you need at school, an online platform or a club that has active members at campuses nationwide can connect you to resources and peers with similar mental health struggles and concerns.

There are hundreds, thousands, or even tens of thousands of students at your school, and millions across the nation. You are not alone. While college is a place for you to challenge yourself and build confidence taking on something new, difficult, and scary, it's also a place that can help you if something gets too overwhelming.

Please take care of your mental health and surround yourself with a good support circle and utilize resources at your university. Poor mental health can compromise your decision-making and lead to destructive behavior when trying to cope with tough situations.

—Ryan, University of California, Los Angeles

Campus-wide Programming

Colleges care about their students. They do! They also care about successfully graduating students on time and how well students do once they enter the workforce or begin postgraduate work. Hence, they try to ease stressors that might hinder your academic performance. There are a lot of distractions in college. Take, for instance, drinking. Even if your campus is dry, schools understand that this can be a dangerous habit for some students, which is why so many reach out to offer support and advice. The following are just some of the campus programs that exist to support you.

Orientation

It used to be that orientation was just a boring info-dump about the credits you'd need to graduate, and many still treat it as a task to quickly check off in order to get to class registration. Times have changed, however, and we urge you to not to zone out or click through to another tab during your orientation.

Schools have crafted a more well-rounded orientation process that aims not only to outline the academic process, but to also prepare students for external situations that may adversely affect them. For instance: learning how to maintain your personal comfort zone when you're being pressured to drink or what to do if you're feeling unsafe at a party. General information like this can be really useful for giving you some context and pointing you in the right direction should you need mental health support.

Orient Yourself

Take a look at your orientation materials or your school's website. Name two resources you find interesting or didn't know were available before. How might this information be helpful?

_____

_____

Student Outreach

The role of student outreach is to connect with students, better understand their needs, and support them by providing resources and referrals. Your student portal account may have a survey, a referral page, or a link to set up an appointment with outreach to get you connected. Student outreach will link you to campus, local community resources, and national organizations for a variety of topics such as economic hardship, sexual assault, and mental health support. These online portals can connect you with everything from housing assistance programs to support groups, so make sure you keep student outreach in mind should you need any of these services.

The state of your mental health is an indicator of what is and isn't working out in your life, so listen to it instead of trying to keep it quiet so that you can (eventually and at your own pace) make decisions that will benefit you in the long run. Reach out to people in your community and at your school. Let someone you trust know what you're going through so that they can be there for you as support while you're going through your struggles. We are all going through our struggles in our different ways, and we can be there to support each other. When you're ready to open up about it, let someone help and support you while you heal. It's okay to ask for help.

—Chloe, Irvine Valley College

Awareness Campaigns

If orientation is the starting point of your educational marathon, then awareness campaigns are the checkpoints found along the course that provide you with fuel and cheer you on to pick up your pace and get back into the race. Checkpoints are speaker series, workshops, health fairs, and online mental health screenings that help you identify or cope with the source of negative feelings. During college, most students will have to deal with something that affects their academics or mental health, or just inhibits their ability function. It's helpful to be reminded that your university hears and supports you.

Guest Speakers

Think about having your very own TED Talk right on campus, giving you access to experts providing tips and insights on something that you really needed to hear. Most colleges have way more resources than your high school, so don't let bad memories of assemblies keep you from at least giving your college's events a chance. As schools continue to recognize the importance of mental health, they are more likely to spend the big bucks to bring in notable speakers and alumni to speak to this cause.

For more free content, visit PrincetonReview.com

Workshops

Workshops are an interactive way to address a mental health topic and engage with a speaker and your peers. This isn't at all a knock against the ability of guest speakers to be totally inspirational! But workshops are often more focused, and are particularly of use to those who want to engage with a speaker and peers, or who want to immediately put the tips and tools being shared into practice.

Fairs

For those who may feel bored by a lecture or intimidated by a group workshop, fairs are a good way to just blend in. You can walk around at your own leisure, grabbing pamphlets as you please. You can also sample from a wider range of representatives at once, which can help you to find the type of organization that best helps you.

Support

Mark Your Calendar

Search on your college's calendar of events or go directly to their counseling page and search keywords such as speakers, fairs, or workshops. Pick an event to attend and mark it on your calendar. Fill in your answer to the question below.

What do you hope to get out of this event? Why is it important for you to listen to this particular topic?

_____

_____

_____

Monthly Wellness Themes

Themes help to provide focus and direction to the speakers, workshops, and fairs being offered by the school, making sure that all aspects of mental health get some form of coverage over the course of a year. (For instance, September, which is National

Suicide Prevention Month, isn't the only month in which you'll find resources, but having it on the calendar helps to normalize the conversation around it and bring some extra attention to those who might otherwise have been unaware of services. Events might include a interview with a specialist on the campus radio station or free counseling sessions for students during that month, so stay tuned. Additionally, stay vocal: if there's a theme you think would be beneficial to your school, you should propose it! Not only will these monthly themes help you become a more aware and better-equipped individual, but the programming can help you feel confident in your ability to take charge of your mental health.

My Month of Mental Health Awareness

Activity

Pick your own monthly topic that you want to prioritize. You can choose one from the list below or come up with your own.

- ☐ Digital Safety

- ☐ Building Connections

- ☐ Substance Misuse Prevention

- ☐ Healthy Relationships

- ☐ Academic Support

- ☐ Grief and Loss

- ☐ LGBTQ+ Community

Write the month in the calendar and set one relevant goal you hope to achieve that month. Assign a new action you can take each week that month to help you reach your goal and improve your overall well-being.

Month:						
Theme:						
Goal:						
SUN	MON	TUES	WED	THURS	FRI	SAT
☐	☐	☐	☐	☐	☐	☐
Week 1 Action:						
☐	☐	☐	☐	☐	☐	☐
Week 2 Action:						
☐	☐	☐	☐	☐	☐	☐
Week 3 Action:						
☐	☐	☐	☐	☐	☐	☐
Week 4 Action:						

Support

Campus-Organized Support

Remember, mental health is an umbrella term for a wide range of conditions that affect your mood, thinking, and behavior. Being in college means you have access to organizations, which means you have a ton of resources at your fingertips. However, not all resources are meant for all conditions. That's where these organizations can help. Often focused on specific mental health topics, or at least well-versed in what's out there, these organizations can help you match the resource you need to your mental health concern. Plus, they're a great source for advocacy, spreading awareness, and support. Here are the types of organizations you will likely encounter.

Student-led Organizations

Student-led organizations differ most from their campus-wide coun-terparts in their specificity. They don't have to work for all students, and so can instead focus on one or two accommodations. They're also run by your peers, which means there tends to be a more familiar atmosphere; you're not talking to a paid expert, but rather working through your issues right along with others who might be doing the same. This is particularly helpful when it comes to destig-matizing certain types of aid, as these groups are more likely to know what you're going through.

Mental Health Clubs

Mental health clubs, while not the same as support groups, work to promote mental health awareness and education within your college community. One of their main missions is to develop an ongoing space for undergrads to discuss mental health topics without stigma. As a group, these club members can do a lot for visibility of mental health resources on campus by leading projects that further their missions.

Active Minds

Active Minds is a nonprofit organization with over 550 student-led clubs on college campuses nationwide. They represent a supportive community of peers ready to discuss mental health issues such as anxiety and depression and also spread awareness throughout campus through events like trivia nights and fundraisers. While they raise awareness and host events, but more importantly, they are a group of individuals who are open and understanding in regards to mental health. Not all meetings are heavy, by the way. You still reap the benefits of a club, attending social events, connecting with others, fostering friendships, and coming together for a common goal, but you get the added bonus of feeling safe discussing mental health in your community.

National Alliance on Mental Illness (NAMI)

The National Alliance on Mental Illness (NAMI) is housed on a number of campuses. They are student-led and have a mission to raise mental health awareness, educate the community, advocate for more support resources, and help students. NAMI clubs are a part of a larger national movement and members also have the opportunity to work with students from peer institutions. Visit https://www.nami.org/home for more information.

Support

Keeping up your mental health is extremely important in college and that's for reasons beyond avoiding burnout, grades, etc. College is where you will meet people that will influence the rest of your life and you will make choices that can lead you down certain paths. Poor mental health can compromise your decision-making and can lead to destructive behavior when trying to cope with tough situations. Please take care of your mental health and surround yourself with a good support circle; utilize resources at your university if you need more help. Enjoy college as much as possible but establish good habits early on, it will make your life so much easier later in your college career.

—Brandon, University of Colorado, Boulder

Peer Counselors

Peer counselors can be a quick, accessible line of defense, especially if there's a waiting list to visit the counseling center. Peer counselors undergo training by faculty or counseling professionals and are equipped to refer you to appropriate resources depending on your needs. Peer counselors can be in a student club, work in the counseling centers, and they often put on events and fundraisers to raise mental health awareness. Let's say you're struggling with a mental health concern and are intimidated by your professor, who is the head of a 300-person class. You can barely talk to him about a research paper, let alone the vulnerability of a mental health issue. Peer counselors not only have lived through similar experiences, but also have tools to be able to support you in advocating for yourself. Oftentimes they can be upperclassmen so you also get tips on what to expect and maybe hear about these students' own personal experiences, helping you feel a little less alone.

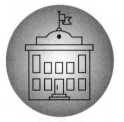

COLLEGE SPOTLIGHT

Hamilton College's peer-counseling program allows students to access free, online appointments with trained peer counselors. Students can read biographies, get to know peer counselors, and easily make an appointment (including on the weekend) with a trusted peer. The counselors provide a safe, non-judgmental space, offer resources, guidance, and referrals for any counseling beyond their area of expertise. Students can work with the same peer counselor throughout their college experience, building a strong relationship, or simply chat with a peer when in need.

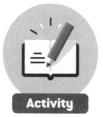

Compare and Contrast

Activity

Pick two mental health organizations you want to try out. Compare and contrast the two, identifying what makes them unique, effective, and possibly a right fit for you.

Think about the following fields to help you complete the diagram:

- Events and Activities

- Mission and Focus

- Members

- Campus and Community Involvement

- Effectiveness & Commitment Level

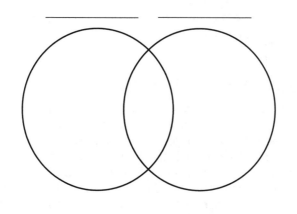

National Organizations

National organizations have the power to connect you with thousands of students nationwide. So, if you feel unheard on a small campus, or if you want mental health resources to support you long after you've graduated, a national organization is a way to achieve that. It's your web of connections spanning beyond campus.

Jed Foundation (Health Programming)

The Jed Foundation is a well-known organization that brings mental health programming to students, including help with life skills, substance abuse, suicide prevention and awareness, and online resources. It's an organization that helps students, but it can also help with life's transition as a young adult. What's different about a powerhouse like the Jed Foundation, is that it brings programming and tools that also connect you to mental health associations and services like ULifeline, discussed below. The Jed Foundation offers dedicated information to fraternities and sororities, allowing students to benefit directly from their resources and utilize them in Greek life. Greek life can bring its own challenges. Seize the Awkward is one of Jed Foundation's campaigns that can help you have mental health conversations with friends, which might feel completely awkward or uncomfortable, especially if you're a part of a larger social group focused primarily on fun.

ULifeline (Health Screenings)

Mental health screenings and daily check-ins can help you monitor your moods over time, which can be incredibly useful in determining when it's time to get some help. ULifeline is an online resource for college mental health where you can access a self-evaluator tool with a questionnaire for depression, anxiety, substance misuse, and eating disorders. Created by the Jed Foundation, the tool connects with your university, so you're directly linked to referrals and resources tailored to where you are. The facts tab lists signs and symptoms for various mental health concerns and provides next steps based on your needs. A "get help now" section directly links you to 24/7 support in a crisis.

Half Of Us (Online Video Libraries)

Let's say you just don't feel like you're connecting with your university as a whole or just aren't ready to open up to a friend. Online video libraries give you a window into others struggling with similar issues, all accessible from your phone or your dorm. Half of Us is one online library packed with videos of celebrities and students sharing their personal experiences with mental health issues and substance abuse, as well as helpful tips. In a testimonial style, celebrities share their mental health challenges from early on in their lives. They discuss about warning signs and symptoms and share how they got help and how they are coping now. Videos also include quick two- to three-minute cartoon vignettes with everything from roommate drama to feeling overloaded.

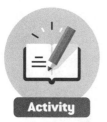

Activity

Evaluate Your Choices

Make note of the type of mental health topics, resources, and issues you are passionate about. Then, get online and evaluate one program to see if their goals align with yours.

Self-Evaluation

■ What mental health topic(s) am I passionate about?

_____

_____

■ What are my goals while participating in a mental health organization?

_____

_____

Support

- Are there any deal breakers (time commitment, mission, etc.) that would prevent me from participating in a national organization?

_____

_____

Organization Evaluation

In the chart below, rate your impression of the organization you've researched, with 1 for strongly disagree and 5 for strongly agree.

This organization's mission aligns with my own.

    ○ 1 ○ 2 ○ 3 ○ 4 ○ 5

This organization would benefit my mental health.

    ○ 1 ○ 2 ○ 3 ○ 4 ○ 5

I could accomplish the things I want to with this organization.

    ○ 1 ○ 2 ○ 3 ○ 4 ○ 5

I have the time to commit to this organization.

    ○ 1 ○ 2 ○ 3 ○ 4 ○ 5

This organization has kind and accepting members.

    ○ 1 ○ 2 ○ 3 ○ 4 ○ 5

This organization is well-organized.

    ○ 1 ○ 2 ○ 3 ○ 4 ○ 5

This organization is inclusive of all types of people.

    ○ 1 ○ 2 ○ 3 ○ 4 ○ 5

This organization would improve my college experience.

    ○ 1 ○ 2 ○ 3 ○ 4 ○ 5

Do you want to attend a call-out meeting for this organization?

Circle: **Yes**   or   **No**

It doesn't matter which type of support program you choose, so pick one that resonates with and fulfills you. Just make sure the one(s) you choose provide an outlet for any negative emotions and can act as a sounding-board for talking through anything you might need help with, from academics to finances to peer relationships and mental health concerns.

REFLECTION

If you could suggest one event for campus mental health programming, what would it be and why?

_____

_____

_____

What types of campus-organized resources (peer counselors, mental health clubs, etc.) are currently available to you? Which one do you feel you could most benefit from? List 2–3 steps you can take to get involved.

_____

_____

_____

How would you describe the presence of national mental health organizations on your campus? In what ways would a national organization benefit you?

_____

_____

_____

CHAPTER 3

Learning Environment

This chapter is all about ensuring that you've got the right learning environment—class size, professors, subjects, schedule—to fit your needs. It will identify the various academic offerings found across colleges, and help you pair them up to best suit your learning styles, so that you feel at ease with (rather than in dread of) your courses. You'll learn to navigate your curriculum and find empowerment in course selection. You'll identify your strengths and blind spots in the classroom and, from there, discover strategies for advocating for your needs.

As if your general education class, History of Medieval Weapons, weren't difficult enough, you're stuck in the middle of a massive 300-person lecture hall. The professor isn't just hard to see, he's hard to hear, and two students behind you keep quietly cracking jokes. You're doing your best to focus, but you lose track of what the teacher's talking about, and when you raise your hand to ask a follow-up, you're sternly reminded that there will be no stopping for questions until the end of the class, if there's time. The notes you're taking aren't making any sense, and you're feeling as if you're falling further and further behind.

You just got off the phone with your family. Your dad has lost his job, and your parents are having trouble managing everything on top of taking care of your younger siblings. As the eldest, you feel a responsibility to step up and try to help support your family and you're miles away trying to figure out what to do. If you take the term off and go back home, you'll be behind in credits. And the thought of taking on another loan to cover an extra semester leaves you feeling anxious and defeated. You're distracted in class and you feel guilty having fun with your friends knowing what's going on back home. You know your family needs your help, but you feel helpless trying to figure out a plan that doesn't derail all the work you've done.

The quarter system is a beast. You're used to your high school schedule with longer semesters, and the idea of turning around work in 10 weeks seems daunting. You're a procrastinator at heart, and while you usually aren't worried about completing your workload, this time it's different. The new class structures are different, you feel distracted, and pushing off your class work just adds more anxiety.

Introduction

Placing yourself in the right classes and the right learning environment can have a big impact on your academics. If you feel completely bored, misunderstood, or cannot handle the work, it will reflect on your overall achievement, not to mention take a toll on you mentally. You have the ability to choose classes, work with advisors, and seek out immersive, engaging academic opportunities that suit your learning styles and needs, leaving you more at ease, rather than feeling dread when it comes to academics.

Depending on which school you attend, your university will offer a number of courses, majors, pathways, and academic opportunities. As a student it is important to know the tools that will allow you to maximize those offerings. Having to include prerequisites and general education requirements in your schedule or having to pick your courses after those with more seniority doesn't mean that you can't have some autonomy in crafting your schedule. You can still determine which classes you take and when, and you can even get creative in fulfilling requirements with more intriguing courses. College is an opportunity to find yourself and explore your strengths, and learning how to balance courses that challenge you, advance you, and refresh you is a skill that will also pay off post-graduation.

Planning your schedule can sometimes feel daunting; there is a lot of balancing time slots and selecting or avoiding certain professors. But ask yourself how much more stressful your semester will be if you just choose courses at random. Do you really want a whole day of lectures or an early morning workshop all the way on the other end of campus?

Learning Environment

The School Year

Each year in college may look a little different, whether you're a first-year managing a quarter system you've never faced or have your first study abroad experience and still want to stay on track toward graduating on time. The school year itself is the calendar you live by. It provides the bigger picture that will drive your monthly goals and daily priorities and determine how you structure your classes. Some years may be more stressful than others, but as you approach each year, you have control over choosing classes and making plans that leave you supported and still challenged, so you're staying afloat.

Semester Structure

The semester structure lends itself to a more traditional school year, much like the one you might have had in high school, with 15-week periods beginning in late August and ending in May, broken up by a winter and summer break.

Pros

Full semesters provide students with a longer period of support. You'll have more time to get to know your professor and adapt to their style, and with a semester ahead of you, the feeling of finals and projects might not sneak up as fast. Classes tend to be shorter, as you won't have to compress as much material into a shorter number of weeks, and your homework will be more spread out, which can help to provide ease in planning your assignments. If something personal or medical crops up, it will likely be easier for you to catch up on anything you've missed.

Cons

If you're a student who loves to procrastinate, a semester's worth of projects, especially for classes that rely on finals and exams rather than multiple assignments, can easily snowball into an incredibly stressful December. If there's a class you aren't doing well in, you're in it for the long haul. This could allow you some time for strategies, but it can also leave you feeling a bit stuck.

Quarterly Structure

In a quarter structure, you're looking at 10-week sessions held in the fall, winter, spring, and typically an optional summer session.

Pros

Additional terms mean that you're likely to be taking fewer classes simultaneously—three or four, as opposed to five or six. This can help students to focus a little more clearly on individual classes, and to do a deeper dive within each. If you're looking to figure out your major, this can be helpful. If you're not loving the teacher, you won't have them for as long. Shorter breaks may seem initially like a drag, but in practice, it can help to keep you in a studying mindset if you're one of those students who finds it difficult to jump back into classes after a long break.

Cons

If you do have a class you're not faring well in, you have less time to form academic strategies and you will need to act fast. If you're someone who needs more time adjusting and organizing your schedule, the jumps between terms may feel quick and a bit overwhelming. If you're someone who really wants to get to know your professors, you'll need to connect with them quicker and early on, which might make you anxious. Internships traditionally align themselves with a semester system, so you'll need to work with an advisor or a faculty member to help you creatively find experiences that boost your resume and fit your schedule.

Studying Abroad

Studying abroad can be an incredible experience, whether you're part of a spring break program or a year-long endeavor. Imagine eating tapas in Spain at 10:00 P.M. because the entire country is still awake, or strolling through an art exhibit, reviewing works from the late 1700s. Studying abroad can bring a sense of confidence and self-growth you might not find at home. Why? Your exposure to diverse and new backgrounds widens your perspective. Although you have guidance from your university, you still are left to navigate a foreign country, with language barriers and new accommodations and customs. It can be a bit overwhelming at first, especially if traveling abroad has always been glorified. Everyone talks about the fun new experiences, but what about the feelings of homesickness and loneliness? Or culture shock?

Here are a few tips to help you before and during your time abroad:

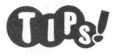

- It is normal to feel homesick, so make sure you keep in touch with a strong support system of friends or family members who can mail you letters (it's nice to have something physical).

- Figure out time zone differences before you depart, and schedule regular phone or video calls that work for both parties.

- If you've previously or are currently struggling with a mental health issue, talk it over with a counselor before you go so that if you're unable to speak with them while abroad, you have some coping strategies and alternatives to fall back on.

- Know that culture shock is temporary. Learning to adapt is part of the experience, so instead of shutting down, continue to soak it in.

- Maintain self-care. Do things that bring you joy. If you ran a lot at home, find a new, safe running route that helps you explore the new area you're in! If you love art, or music, find time to check out new architecture, museums, and festivals in the area.

- Seek out other students who are studying abroad, as you may be able to build a friendship over your common struggles to adapt.

- Bond with locals while abroad as well! Find common ground and use that to take your support system global.

Winter/Summer Classes

Winter and summer classes can be a space for you to tackle one class that you know is going to be a bit harder and that you want to focus your attention on. It can also be a time when you can knock out elective classes that you need to work your way towards upper division coursework or just to fulfill credits. Keep in mind that the terms are traditionally shorter, so if you are focusing on one class that you know is going to be tougher, ensure that you're able to learn the material in a shorter amount of time, and that you have resources available if you need extra help, such as tutoring, or backing off of any responsibilities so that you can to focus solely on the course.

If there is a class that you can take at a local community college, over the summer and it transfers to your institution, you have the opportunity to save money and get through some credits. Note that these classes will primarily be in your lower division classes or any pre-major coursework. Work with an advisor ahead of time to ensure the classes will transfer.

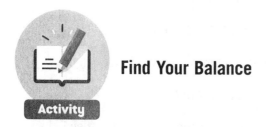

Find Your Balance

Activity

Jot down a list of courses that you are eligible for and interested in taking next semester.

_____

_____

_____

_____

Learning Environment

Ask yourself the following questions for each course. Put an *X* to the left each time you make that choice and a ✔ to the right each time you make that choice.

You believe this class will be

_____ HARD or EASY _____

How have you performed in this subject before?

_____ POORLY or WELL _____

Your main reason for taking this class is for

_____ A REQUIREMENT or PLEASURE _____

You've heard or know this professor is

_____ DIFFICULT or EASY _____

This class is offered at a time of day where you will be

_____ SLEEPY or ALERT _____

If you need help with the course, how many friends have taken or will be taking it?

_____ NONE/ONE or TWO OR MORE _____

Count each check on the left as −1 and each check on the right as +1. Your classes should now all have a value from −6 to +6. As you put together a schedule, try to make sure that the total value of courses is 0 or higher.

Curriculum

Think of your college curriculum as a series of checkpoints, like those you might find in a race—except that this one goes off-and-on for roughly four years. (That's why it's important to take breaks to rehydrate and catch your breath!) In order to graduate, there are a certain number of classes that you must complete.

Core, or general education, courses are those that every student at the school must complete, and these can range from seminars about life skills to writing workshops. Many liberal arts universities, looking to produce well-rounded graduates, require their students to take a few history, math, and science classes, much like high school, but with far more variety within those departments. Some schools that have a particular focus or specialization, like business, are likely to have more core courses within those fields.

Once you've declared a major or minor, that department will provide you with a more specialized curriculum. Instead of general courses, these will be a tiered series of programming, a bit like a layer cake, in which you must complete a certain number of basic 100-level courses in that subject in order to qualify for the intermediate 200-level classes and, eventually, the 300-level programming that you'll need in order to graduate.

Then again, some schools allow students to build their own majors, coming up with an agreed-upon curriculum that satisfies the academic departments who would be conferring that degree. You may also find schools with open curricula, where students can work their way through various areas of study until they find their particular expertise.

Doubling Up and Doubling Over

It is absolutely possible for a single course to fulfill multiple requirements. A good schedule-building exercise is to list everything you need to graduate—total number of credits, number of classes within a specific subject, prerequisites, types of classes—and cross out or adjust this list so that you can see how each new class is moving you toward the finish line.

Learning Environment

This doesn't mean that you shouldn't take a class that you're interested in, but which fulfills few, if any, of your graduation goals. There are, after all, benefits to breaking up the monotony of an all-economics course-load with a film class you feel passionate about, and you never know when studying something seemingly unrelated, like philosophy or psychology, will actually open up a brand-new way of thinking about your chosen career. Switching between heavy and light classes also gives your brain a chance to refresh and, more importantly, introduces you to students outside your major, which is important, as a broader network can lead to additional opportunities down the road. It can be a change of pace and keep you on your toes, and, who knows, it might actually end up being fun, like the Massachusetts Institute of Technology's How to Stage a Revolution class or the Ice Cream Short Course at Pennsylvania State University. Colorado College offers arts and craft courses, and Yale has The Science of Well-Being, one of the university's most popular courses. Why? Perhaps it has something to do with studying happiness and finding tangible ways to increase productivity by incorporating wellness into your routine. Sign me up!

University is your opportunity to explore and try new things and if you only do what you think you like cause that's all you know, you will leave so many doors closed that you didn't even know were a possibility. It's all about pushing yourself outside of your comfort zone to really understand who you are.

—Lucas, University of Western Ontario

Course Cruising

Find one class in the course catalogue that's completely out of your wheelhouse but that you think sounds interesting. Write down the name of the class and what you think it could teach you.

_____

_____

Specialized Programming

Finding ways to tailor your academics can help you in a number of ways. For starters, if you're looking to differentiate yourself from the general student population, finding a specialized program may be the ticket. Specialized programming is just that, specialized. They help you tailor your education to best fit your needs and desired outcomes.

Certificate Programs

Certificate programs are a great way to complement your major while developing and demonstrating your specialized interests. More credits than a minor but less than a major, these interdisciplinary programs offer students ways to diversify their education in a more targeted fashion. Some students even find that their certificate program addresses topics they were interested in but were left out of the curriculum for their major. This is a great choice for students if they're looking to customize their education and stand out to postgraduate programs or future employers.

Honors Cohorts

Honors colleges and programs provide ambitious students with the chance to take a deep dive into some serious academic studies and build strong relationships with faculty members. Honors colleges can be across the college as a whole, within a specific school (like an honors program for the busines school), or even within a department (like the honors program for the English department). Most of these require that you apply for and meet certain standards that are evaluated based on your transcript, resume, recommendations, or writing samples. Once accepted, it opens up access to big research projects, special classes, and more, that will help you to not only stand out among your peers, but make you feel more in control of your academic agenda.

Pre-Professional Tracks

A pre-professional track is tailored to help students with certain career goals in mind, such as law, medicine, or pharmacy. Undergrads enrolled in these programs work with an advisor who

Learning Environment

helps you pick out the best classes, extracurriculars, and activities to help you get into a professional program down the line. They also assist with applications, mock interviews, and more. Just as the professional programs are highly competitive and require a number of prerequisites, so too are pre-professional programs. If you're interested in a field to which this type of specialization is applicable, make sure you're dedicated to putting in your best effort from beginning to end.

Dual Degree Programs

Dual degree programs allow you to complete two very different degrees at once. If you're an undergraduate, the two most common dual degree programs are 1) one that confers two different bachelor's degrees, like a BA and a BS or 2) one that combines a bachelor's with a master's degree, such as a BA/MBA. Students who have very diverse academic interests they want to pursue extensively are a great fit for these programs. Although the workload for this type of coursework can be extremely demanding, in the long run, you spend less time doing both degrees simultaneously.

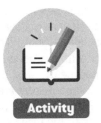

Activity

On The Right Track

Using the prompts on the left, fill in the space on the right to get an idea of how you can focus your area(s) of study given your preferences, strengths, and time available.

Topics

What class subjects do I like?

What do I want to learn more of?

Are there any subjects I'd like to explore? Or, any classes I can add to specialize in my major?

Coursework

What kind of assignments do I prefer?

Do I prefer working in groups or alone?

Am I a self-motivated learner, or do I prefer to have a mentor or guided track?

Do I have a particular career in mind that my coursework is helping me reach?

Timing

How are my time management skills?

Is my class schedule currently set up to meet my long-term goals and stay on track credit-wise?

Using this preliminary brainstorm, head to your school's website or visit your academic advisor and identify one specialization method (dual degree, certificate program, honors college, etc.) that interests you. Explain below why you think it's a good fit and what would be your next step in learning more about it.

Learning Environment

Academic Advisors

Managing all of the various requirements for graduation can be tricky, which is why there are a variety of advisors offering support. Some of these are mandatory resources; you'll have to meet with them in order to get permission to take certain upper-level classes. Here's a list of who to go to for advice in different situations:

Advisor Type	What They Can Do
Department Advisor	• Review your previous coursework (like APs or transferred classes from another college) and let you know what, if any, requirements you've already satisfied. • Provide special permission to take a class in advance of a prerequisite. • Offer guidance in selecting a major. • Provide insight to career outlooks.
Professor	• Review portfolio submissions to permit entry to their class. • Offer research opportunities. • Provide feedback on your research. • Give professional insight into various careers. • Write you a letter of recommendation.
Peer Advisor	• Provide student insight on choosing classes and also experiences with professors. • Provide general information and tips on things like class registration, campus resources, waitlisting classes, and general education classes. • Know the material for classes you'll take and can host study groups. • Help you transition into university life. • Offer academic tips on study skills, time management, etc.

Advisor Type	What They Can Do
General Advisor	• Help you transition into university life. • Build an academic plan. • Help you explore majors based on your interests, strengths, and skills. • Refer you to campus resources such as tutoring, career services, and study abroad offices. • Ensure that you are meeting university requirements and fulfilling appropriate class credits.

Classroom Environment

As you take classes, begin noticing which environments you tend to do better in. You might have to take a large lecture class and find that you feel completely disconnected. You might prefer the small group that meets with a teacher's assistant because it helps you clarify material you missed because it was hard to hear or you just zoned out for a bit and weren't able to ask the professor. You might find that working in a lab helps you better understand the larger concepts because you're able to visualize the problem and literally work through a solution with your hands. Not every class is going to be your favorite. That is completely normal! Gaining a better understanding of the classes you do well in makes it easier to design a schedule chock-full of them.

My preference is large classes that record lectures, but I've found that other types of classes have their own benefits. One of my favorite classes was a small, 30-person class that didn't record their lectures, and I found that I was way more engaged and learning way more than I usually do. I think it's important to be open to different types of classes!

—Yasmine, University of California, Los Angeles

Large Lecture Halls

Large lecture halls, even if you're in a smaller university, can often be a part of your experience, especially in lower division or pre-requisite classes. If it's something completely new to you, it can feel a bit intimidating. Use your class time in the way that works best for you, and don't worry if it looks different than your neighbor's method! You might hate the idea of asking a question in front of all those people, so use the class time to take notes, observe, and listen, and take advantage of professors' office hours or the weekly small-group teaching assistant sessions to ask follow-up questions. Maybe you're a student who needs to listen and absorb information. In this case, see if there are recorded lectures so you can just focus and listen throughout the lecture, writing down larger concepts and filling in the holes after reviewing the recording.

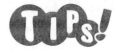

Here are some of our best tips for thriving in a large class:

- Sit where you feel most comfortable: the front row is best for avoiding distractions, but there are other places to sit if you don't want to be right under the professor's eye.

- If you notice the class gets full and finding a seat is harder as class time nears, get to class early, choose your spot, and review your notes or the reading prior to class, or just hang out and sit for a minute.

- Your laptop or phone can be a blessing for taking notes, but a massive distractor if you're shopping or browsing social media. You can put your phone in airplane mode or set a browser extension to block certain websites for the allotted class time.

- If the class is going to be for more than an hour or two, prepare ahead of time by bringing snacks, water, and a charger for your laptop.

- Attend class! It can be really freeing if attendance is never taken. However, that freedom can quickly turn sour if you've banked on trying to learn the material the night before a midterm or final. Go to class. Just go.

Small Discussion-Based Classes

Small discussion-based classes can demand more preparation than showing up to a lecture. When it's a group of ten debating foreign policy, and you've bailed on your reading, it's never a good look. Allow yourself time to check what's needed for the next meeting and prepare. Connect with a peer in the group and use them for accountability. Prepare talking points ahead of time. If you're sitting in a small group, especially if you're not used to it, have a few bullet points of the material or what you'd like to contribute to class. Use them as a guide when you feel a bit lost.

Last, communicate with your professor. In these types of classes, the number of students is so small, and often the classroom is based on discussions and interactions, so it'll be noticed if you're missing! Let the professor know if you'll be absent, obtain any readings and information, and follow up with a peer in the class to review any material prior to the next class meeting.

I haven't quite pinned down my learning style yet, but I have found that the more excited my teacher is, the more I enjoy the class, and smaller class sizes can be better because it's easier to reach out to peers and make friends, or even just convince people to do a study group for a big test.

—*Annabel, Lewis and Clark*

Grading Policies

Every teacher grades their class differently. Some professors put a premium on attendance and class participation. Others give regular assignments that provide you with a steady way of gaining points and tracking your overall progress before a deadline. Some teachers make you put all your eggs in one basket, scoring you based on the results of a few tests or papers, which is great if you like high-stakes assignments, but maybe not the best if you tend to procrastinate.

Grades can be a huge stressor in college, so take the steps to understand your professors' policies and how to communicate with them about your work and grades.

Dropping a Class

At the beginning of each term, record the deadlines to drop a class and adjust your schedule if need be. If last spring you felt egregious and added Genetics and Molecular Biology only to realize it doesn't couple well with your Organic Chemistry, shifting one class to another term and fulfilling an elective credit can help evenly balance your course load. But if you miss the drop deadline, you're left with a "W" for withdrawing on your transcript or paying a fee for a class you end up not taking. Look at your schedule as a whole and assess all the extras that come into play (the makeup of the class, who's teaching it, what extracurricular commitments you have, etc.) and if you realize you've bitten off more than you can chew, pull back. If you do choose to drop a class, be extra cautious and meet with an advisor to make sure your student status and financial aid won't be affected.

Homework Prep

Pick any of your assignments and go through the following exercises to see if you're prepared for class.

Have I taken the steps to understand the material to the best of my abilities and turned in a complete assignment?

- ❏ Read all required material.

- ❏ Answered all questions or completed all required writing.

- ❏ Reviewed previous lecture notes to prepare for the next discussion.

Write down 2–3 concepts you did not understand or questions that you have.

_____

_____

_____

Prepare a response to the question "What did I think about the reading?"

_____

_____

_____

Offer 3–5 talking points that are relevant to the course (main take-aways, related to current events, tied into the course theme, etc.).

_____

_____

_____

_____

_____

Learning Environment

Academic Problems & Coping Strategies

Academics are overwhelming, and it can take a big toll on you mentally. You can meet with advisors, create a beautiful schedule, and still walk away from your first few weeks of class feeling a bit defeated because you're unable to grasp the new concepts or understand the subject matter. It's okay to have classes you don't like, fail an assignment, or even listen to a lecture and feel like it's in a foreign language (when it's not a foreign language course!). Part of growing is feeling uncomfortable. There are strategies to help you manage even the most difficult classes and keep you from falling into the 40% of students who feel that their work is hopeless.

Increased Rigor or Workload

As you progress through your classes, the material will advance. One of the challenges as you grow is understanding the new material, going at a quicker pace, and applying what you've learned in prerequisite classes to advance concepts. The rigor of your classes is meant to challenge you mentally, but it can also leave you a bit drained. This can happen as you get further into your degree course, or when there's a class that's not necessarily your jam, but it's required to fulfill your degree. Sure, it might just be one class, but it can be a real pain mixed in with everything else and leave you frustrated.

How to Cope

The secret to managing increased academic rigor is the same as the secret to getting through a long road trip: pacing. You'll feel a lot less depleted if you know what time of day you're most productive and alert and if you leave room for breaks. As you go through your school day, you're exerting energy and depleting your brain tank. So why would you schedule your hardest class at 2 P.M. if that's the time you usually crash? The lower your tank is, the less capacity you have to focus on the task at hand.

Now think about your overall schedule and where you can prioritize your time to meet the demands of the tough classes. Your class schedule is static, but how you spend your free time is up for consideration. So if you have two hours to study, your priority will be to complete the assignments or readings for your hardest class *first* and then progress to your easier subjects from there. It might feel like a good idea to knock out your easiest class first, gain some confidence, and move forward. But remember, you're still using brain power, whether it feels simple or not, so consider what will use the most of it and do that task first.

Similarly, think about how you spend your weeks. If you're someone who would thrive knocking out all your classes in two or three days, by all means, go for it! But if you need more wiggle room each day, don't trick yourself into thinking you'll be happy overbooking yourself. That would be like committing to do an 18-hour road trip in one day when you know you're exhausted by hour ten. Knowing how you like not only your days, but your weeks paced will prevent burnout and give you the boost of energy you need to tackle increasingly difficult academics.

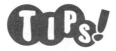

- Limit distractions before you begin. Check notifications and then promptly turn your phone on airplane mode, close all tabs on your browser you do not need, clear any clutter around the table, etc.

- Use a standing desk or give yourself stretch breaks in between sitting down for long periods of time.

- Set up your space before you begin studying by plugging in your devices, having your water/snacks if needed, textbooks out, pencils, computer, etc.

- Adjust the lighting, if you can, or find a space with lighting that appeals to you. This could be a darker room in a library or sunny area outside. Whatever works!

- Find electronics that make things comfier and reduce distractions such as noise-cancelling headphones, a mouse for your laptop, etc.

- Post goals, or write inspirational words to keep you going when you're fried.

Learning Environment

Plan Your Academic Road Trip

In the space below, write down your current or most recent courses and fill up the gas tank with how much effort you'll need to put into each class.

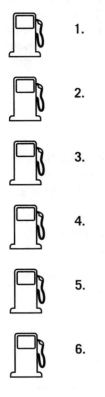

1.

2.

3.

4.

5.

6.

Now, choose one day of the week. First, fill in your classes and extracurricular commitments, and check off the hours of the day that are going toward those.

Then, fill in any assignments (or readings) that you want to get done, and see where there's free time left to get it done. If you can't find time for breaks, take a step back.

Tasks	Day of the week
Classes: _____ _____ _____ _____ **Commitments:** _____ _____ _____ **———————————** **Assignment/Readings:** _____ _____ _____ _____ _____ _____ _____ _____	☐ 8 A.M. ☐ 9 A.M. ☐ 10 A.M. ☐ 11 A.M. ☐ 12 P.M. ☐ 1 P.M. ☐ 2 P.M. ☐ 3 P.M. ☐ 4 P.M. ☐ 5 P.M. ☐ 6 P.M. ☐ 7 P.M. ☐ 8 P.M. ☐ 9 P.M. ☐ 10 P.M. ☐ 11 P.M. ☐ 12 A.M. ☐ 1 A.M.

Learning Environment

Test Anxiety

It's fairly normal to experience some degree of stress leading up to exams, but if you're experiencing an unhealthy amount to where it's hindering learning and consistently hurting your ability to perform on tests, then it's time to get some help. Here are examples of what test/performance anxiety tends to look like:

- Sweating

- Shaking

- Rapid heartbeat

- Dry mouth

- Feeling faint

- Stomach pain/nausea

- Excessively fidgety

- Having a hard time focusing or remembering information

- Feeling helpless in a testing situation

How to Cope

To manage test anxiety, begin with the time leading up to the test. At the beginning of each term, review your syllabi and input all exam dates in your calendar. When you're preparing, allow yourself enough time to learn and absorb the information. Work backwards from the dates in your syllabi and schedule designated time to review new material you're shaky on, as well as time to refresh your memory of older topics or concepts you may have forgotten. Give yourself enough lead time to cover everything you need without overwhelming yourself. As you get closer to test day, particularly the day before an exam, get plenty of sleep, avoid substance use, and eat well. Cramming in another hour of reading at 11:00 P.M. the night before will only backfire. At that point, sleep will be a better use of your time.

On the morning of the exam, allow yourself plenty of time to get to class. If you're already worried about doing well on the midterm, running late and not having a moment to get situated will only make it worse. When the exam begins, read through instructions carefully, review how much time you have, and take slow, deep breaths if you find any anxiety creeping in. You can also squeeze your fists under your desk, refocus your energy, and release, letting it all go, physically allowing your body and mind to relax. Lastly, avoid getting caught in the perfectionist trap and setting unrealistic standards for yourself. Ask yourself how you would help a friend battling with test anxiety. The kind words you'd share with a friend are the same kind words you want to use for yourself! You've worked hard, and one exam is just that: one exam. It's not your entire degree, nor is it determining the rest of your life. If your anxiety is getting to the point where it's crippling, causing you to miss class or consistently affecting your grades, it's time to talk to someone. A counselor, your professor, or a trusted advisor are all places to start.

Falling Behind

What if you're behind in classes and your books are left untouched or that Google doc that was supposed to be your first research paper is still blank? Or how about neglecting to finish the calc assignment because you keep getting the same questions wrong and can't figure out why, so you just shut your laptop, telling yourself you'll do it later. Everyone has a class they dread or struggle with, and the feeling of falling behind can cause a lot of mental stress, not to mention leaving you drained, because what was supposed to be a productive homework session has turned into frustrating hours of not getting through the work you don't understand.

How to Cope

First, figure out the root problem that's causing you to fall behind. Is it your lack of time management? Is a concept hard to grasp, or are the demands of the course in general overloading you? Next, find a resource that can help you. Your university has vast resources to help support your academic needs (remember those advisors we listed earlier? Check with them!). Most of the time, there's something that's a great fit for your situation, and you just never knew it was there or that you needed it in the first place.

Things you're familiar with, like tutoring, are widely available, but really do your research and get specific as to which center will help you best, such as a writing lab, a department tutor, or even a peer tutor who has taken (or is currently taking) the class and can walk you through assignments. Reaching out to those who are there to support you academically—like professors and advisors—can introduce you to services involving technology, study groups, and more.

I Need Accommodations

What if you have trouble presenting in front of people. You hate it, and even though it's something you know you'll have to work through for future class presentations, right now it's bringing you anxiety, crippling anxiety to the point where you dread class. Alternatively, what if you struggle with dyslexia and college level reading is a huge jump from high school, and now you're not sure about your comprehension level. There might be something affecting a number of students where the learning environment needs to be adjusted, or something personally affecting you like the death of a friend or financial strain, where the demands can overtake your academic responsibilities and you're forced to adjust accordingly. Asking for accommodations, no matter what you're dealing with, is something that can be very stressful, but is essential to making the learning process less taxing.

How to Cope

It's important to let the necessary people—like counselors, advisors, and professors—know what's going on so they can help you. There are structures in place to make college a safe place to ask for accommodations. Advocate for yourself! You are your biggest champion. If you don't ask, the door closes right then and there. Here are some of the top things you can do to advocate for yourself.

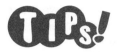

- Communicate. Let the appropriate people know about arrangements you need or have set up.

- Know your strengths and weaknesses and areas that you need more help with before you feel frustrated or misunderstood.

- Find a community of tutors, mentors, academic support offices, etc., who can help you adjust your accommodations or intervene if needed.

- Know your rights to accommodations and support if you have a learning disability or a diagnosed mental health issue.

- Be confident in yourself! Believe in your ability to succeed in college and treat slipups as learning opportunities and move on.

If you have a learning difference, reach out to your school's academic office and disability services to see what accommodations are available. Do this as early in the semester as possible, before any potential issues manifest, as you will likely need to provide the department with documentation. There may also be additional programs and services that you can register for, like getting recordings provided to you (in a class that does not normally offer them) or having captions and class notes provided to you to aid in your studies.

Learning Environment

COLLEGE SPOTLIGHT

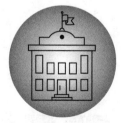

Students with learning differences and attention challenges can apply to be a part of the University of Arizona's Strategic Alternative Learning Techniques (SALT) Center and receive academic support with the help of a student support specialist. Specialists work with students on everything from time management and creating academic and personal goals to fostering learning strategies and developing individual learning plans for students.

If your school does not already have the resources you need, don't give up! Communicate as clearly as possible what would help you, as the school may be able to develop those services or put you in touch with peers, counselors, advisors, or professors who may be able to provide them, on a case-by-case basis.

COLLEGE SPOTLIGHT

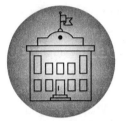

The University of Denver's Learning Effectiveness Program offers similar programming and models its services after self-advocacy, self-accountability, self-determination, and self-awareness, helping students not only to achieve academically, but personally and socially, as well. Students have the opportunity to participate in the Journey to Empowerment Through Transition (JETT) experience, where they're provided with guidance and skills to transition and cope with university life effectively. Students gain resources and support to help prepare for choosing classes, assimilating on campus, navigating academic, social, and developmental tasks involved with the college experience, and planning for change in the future regarding career-making decisions.

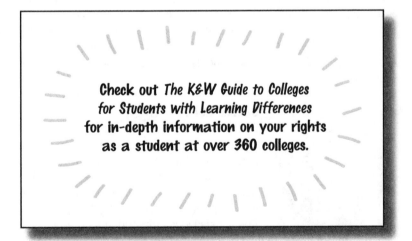

Check out *The K&W Guide to Colleges for Students with Learning Differences* for in-depth information on your rights as a student at over 360 colleges.

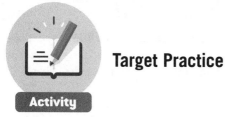

Target Practice

In the bullseye, write the biggest problem you're currently facing in regards to academics. In each ring, write down possible solutions. The ones on the outside are the easiest, most temporary fixes, while the ones moving toward the center are harder but ultimately most effective. Be specific.

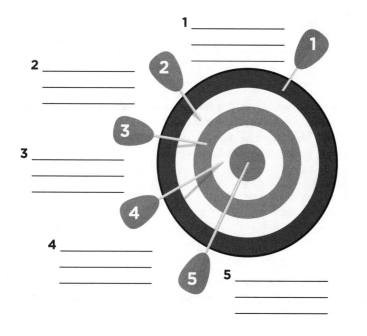

Learning Environment

REFLECTION

What's one thing you can do to better manage the school year?

_____

_____

How do you feel about the makeup of your academic coursework thus far? Are their topics or concepts you're hoping to learn more about in the coming semester(s)? Explain.

_____

_____

_____

When was the last time you took a class and did incredibly well? What did you like about the course, how was the material delivered, and if you had the opportunity to take other classes with similar styles, why would it be helpful to you?

_____

_____

_____

How confident are you advocating for yourself in an academic setting? What steps can you take to be more comfortable doing so?

_____

_____

CHAPTER 4

Exercise

In this chapter you will learn about different forms of exercise, whether you're training for strength or endurance. You will also be more tuned in to the various student organizations, programs, and facilities on college campuses that may be of help. There will be opportunities for you to check in with where you are currently and create future goals to stay on track. Lace up your shoes, grab some water, and let's go.

Finals are just around the corner, and you realize you've sunk into a bit of a work-heavy routine. It's gotten so bad that you realize you're eating dinner at your desk while you do your homework, and to make up for the lack of movement, you've started pacing while brushing your teeth just to make your step count seem less...sad. Those rare times when you finally do catch a break, you're too exhausted to even stand at the foosball table, and you don't want to do anything but plop down on your lounge's couch and watch TV. It seems there's no time or energy to get your body moving.

After years of hard work, you're finally a starter on your varsity team, but now you've got to do even more to prove yourself and keep your position. You've been drilling outside of regular hours, practicing in the quad after the sun sets, and you've also got a part-time job at a local warehouse helping to restock goods. You thought you were in good shape, but lately, you've been starting to feel like you're pushing it too far, and soaking in an ice bath isn't doing it like it used to. You know you need to focus on recovery, but you can't stop now—can you?

Whether it's too much exercise or not enough, your body is calling out for a change, and your mind keeps stressing out about it. *A nice relaxing walk? No thanks. I can hardly cram in all of my homework, studying, and activities as is.* You're going to have to give *somewhere*, especially now that the soreness is making it harder to focus during exams. You've seen your grades start to slip. That tight calf muscle, that knot in your back—if you don't find a happy medium, you're going to be ex-exercise.

Introduction

A majority of students across the country—56%, according to some reports—are faced with overwhelming stressors. Between a full academic calendar and the expectation to succeed in your classes without falling behind, you're also constantly being cautioned not to miss out on the college experience. How are you supposed to manage it all? Believe it or not, routine exercise might be your answer. Did you know that students who consistently utilized the recreation and fitness facilities in their first and second years had higher GPAs than their peers who did not? Not only did they have higher GPAs, but they also tended to have more credits completed on average. We'd all like to graduate on time with a high GPA!

Incorporating this healthy habit into your life will not only help you cope with the stressors of college, but it can build a strong foundation for years to come. One of the biggest challenges you face in college is learning how to "adult." You have increasingly difficult workloads, are trying to build a social life while managing your health, stress, and finances, and you have to figure out what kind of career you're interested in. Your responsibilities and to-do list seem endless. Looking for a way to manage stress or improve your mood? How about learning to build a routine? Physical activity has you covered on both fronts. Exercise has the ability to improve your mood and kick negative effects of stress to the curb.

You don't have to be a Division 1 athlete to incorporate physical activity into your life. There are tons of exercise varieties for you to pick and choose from. Exercise can be broken down into the following four groups: endurance, strength, balance, and flexibility. We'll go more in depth into each of these categories later in the chapter, but each type of physical activity benefits your body and mental health in some way.

There's no better time to learn what workouts you like than your college years when you have access to your school's facilities. Most schools have some sort of recreation center with at least your standard gym equipment (weights, track), but many also offer various classes and specialized resources. You might find you love swimming laps in the pool or waking up for a spin class that meets every Monday. Some students find that they like to combine their fitness routine and social lives and join an intramural or club team. There are a wide variety of organized and recreational activities to think about, from basketball and flag football to battleship and wallyball. Don't be afraid to try something new! It's worth at least seeing what's offered and which exercise routine sticks. If you need more accountability, grab a couple of friends, and set a time to meet. Students who have peers who will work out and take classes with them are often more likely to keep it up.

Sometimes working out on campus isn't possible, whether that's because your school doesn't have the facility or activity you want, the gym is closed when you're free, or you just need a change of scenery to get motivated. When that's the case, get creative and look at what's available in your surrounding community. Keep your eye out for local offerings at community gyms or fitness centers and think about events, like 5Ks, that might seem interesting to you. You can also go it solo by utilizing the natural workout "rooms" of a park or preserve, where you might be able to get in some hiking or climbing. (And when we say "go solo," you can still check with your campus to see if they rent any gear.)

When all else fails, you can take exercise into your own hands. Literally. There are a number of free or low-fee apps that you can download and use from the comfort of your dorm room or on the go. You can choose from live or pre-recorded classes, filtering by the amount of time and equipment that you have available, while still getting activities tailored to your individual body weight.

Spend some time finding the perfect mix of activities for your lifestyle and needs. Having a clear idea of what exercise you prefer, what is accessible, and how to incorporate it will help you stay consistent. There's no one perfect routine for everyone, so as you try new exercises, pay attention to the ones you like. Not everyone loves the idea of running, but you might really like quick 20-minute workouts in your dorm. The goal is consistency. Why? Because that's where you begin to reap the rewards like that higher GPA, or at least a clear mind at the end of a long day.

Types of Exercise

You hear about fitness across mediums, from your doctors to exercise influencers on social media—even your friends might talk about it! As you may have noticed from your interactions with these people, there are about a million and one ways to be active.

By all means, be encouraged to get active, but don't just jump into a heavy routine. Pushing your body too hard can lead to negative results, so as you read through these possible activities, start slow and consider consulting with your physician or an on-campus fitness specialist.

Endurance

Endurance exercises, or aerobics, increase your breathing and heart rate. It gets your body moving, your heart pumping, and your endorphins flowing. Endurance workouts have the ability to burn calories and keep your circulatory system, heart, and lungs healthy. The American Heart Association recommends at least 150 minutes of moderate to intense aerobic activity a week, which equates to about 20 minutes a day, or 30 minutes Monday through Friday (Yes, you can still keep your weekend). You can hop on an elliptical in the student gym, go for a walk/run around campus, swim, and hike. If team sports are your thing, join a pickup game of volleyball or basketball in an open gym. Maybe there is a dance class that fits with your schedule, or a set of bleachers you can use for running up and down steps when there aren't any games going on. These are all great options!

Exercise

Find what works for you. Start small and get creative with endurance exercises, even if that's walking across campus rather than hopping on the bus or taking the stairs instead of the elevator up to your fifth-floor class. This is a great way to gradually increase the level of activity. Every person is different, so it can be helpful to create a routine and keep track of your progress. For example, maybe you begin walking a half-mile three times a week. Then after a few weeks, maybe you walk for a mile, or jog for half a mile and then walk the rest to complete a full mile. As you build your strength, you'll find yourself breathing easier and getting stronger. And if you end up wanting to train for a marathon, well, you might find a class or a group on campus to help you do just that.

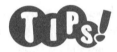

Here's a three-pronged approach to endurance that you can work into your workout.

1. Warm up. Before each session, warm up for five to ten minutes with a brisk walk or jump-rope, for example, increasing blood flow to your muscles and revving your cardiovascular system.

2. Conditioning. At your own pace, work up to at least 30 minutes of cardio a day. By increasing your heart rate, you're increasing your aerobic capacity and ability to breathe easier.

3. Cool-down. You're done! Now cool down for five to ten minutes by stretching your muscles, from your legs, to your arms, and throughout your entire body, allowing your heart rate and muscles to return to normal.

Strength

Maybe you already feel pretty comfortable with lifting weights, or perhaps the idea of lifting barbells feels barbaric. Regardless of your style, adding strength to your workout can be really helpful for things like building muscle, toning, and overall health. Weight training doesn't require superhuman power. In fact, you can incorporate bodyweight exercises and even add small resistance bands to a simple routine and increase your strength ability. Simple moves that require no equipment all, such as squats, lunges, and pushups all count as strength exercises. You can add weights as you feel more powerful and in control while keeping proper form, meaning you're not throwing a dumbbell up in the air only to find you've thrown out your shoulder. Everyone has a different level, so as you begin adding strength, note which weights, or how many bodyweight reps, you are completing in a set.

Check to see what the gym at your university offers and ask for help if you need it. There's no shame in having someone who works at the rec center show you how to use the machines or give you a few exercises. You might find a free consultation where a trainer can show you some simple moves in one visit or get some advice from the physical therapy or exercise science department. If you're feeling super intimidated, you can try simple moves in your dorm that are quick and efficient.

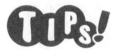

Ways to improve your strength training routine:

- Take a class and learn proper form
- Do more sets and repetitions
- Add more weight (safely!)
- Target muscle groups
- Create a routine that fits with your schedule
- Keep track of your progress

Flexibility and Balance

Flexibility and balance can reduce your risk of injury and improve your posture and mobility. It can also be a great workout. Think about rolling out your yoga mat and getting into a nice flow. Your phone is in your bag in the corner, in airplane mode, and you have 40 minutes of core work and stretching that will leave you invigorated. Yoga and Pilates are a couple of forms of exercises that increase your flexibility and also your strength! You can incorporate stretching into your workout routine as a warm-up or a cool down, or simply between classes if you've been sitting all day in lectures. You can even stretch in your dorm before you head off for your day. Up your balance game with core workouts. Ab workouts, like tree-poses in yoga, can all add to a stronger core, helping you increase strength. And, let's face it, when you've been sitting in a chair all day with your shoulders hunched, something as simple as lying on your back and stretching out your entire body can be a game changer.

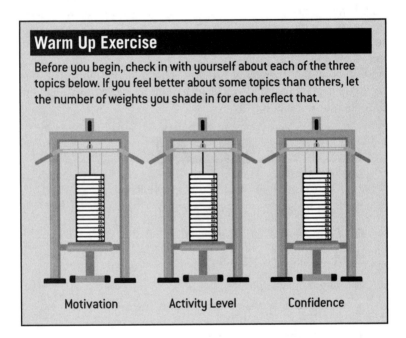

Warm Up Exercise

Before you begin, check in with yourself about each of the three topics below. If you feel better about some topics than others, let the number of weights you shade in for each reflect that.

Motivation   Activity Level   Confidence

Access to Exercise Facilities

Hopefully, you're feeling a bit inspired to break out a sweat and try something new. There are lots of places to look on campus, off campus, and even from the comfort of your own room or on the go. Dive in!

This or That

In this quick heads-up, circle your immediate preferences:

1. Exercise: Class / Alone
2. Activity: Indoor / Outdoor
3. Sports: Team / Solo
4. Workout: Long / Short
5. Workout: Morning / Evening
6. Workout: Spin / HIIT
7. Workout: Weights and Machines / No Equipment

On-Campus Facilities

There are really cool spaces on college campuses that will allow you to thrive by supporting you physically. Depending on where you attend college, there are a few types of facilities generally accessible that provide you with a range of activities to choose from. You can easily search a university's health facilities online or take a tour and find out information such as:

- how many locations they have
- hours of operation
- how accessible it is to the general student population
- schedules of class offerings
- rates, if applicable

Ask around or see for yourself what the facilities' busiest times are. If you're more likely to ditch a workout because the room is full and it feels a bit intimidating, try a different time. As you explore facilities and workouts, be open to trying new things, and if something doesn't work, check out a new class or a different area. Building a routine takes some trial and error, but as a college student, you

Exercise

most likely have access so some incredible facilities and if it's included in your tuition, take advantage!

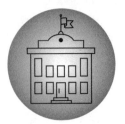

COLLEGE SPOTLIGHT
Don't forget to check your course cata-logue for courses that have fitness compo-nents or are just outright gym classes. You can find some pretty unique opportunities that'll keep you fit and teach you new skills. Pepperdine University, for example, offers an introduction to surfing class. Cornell has tree-climbing, and the University of Utah has a backcountry skiing course.

CHAARG (Student Organizations)

CHAARG (Changing Health, Attitudes, and Actions to Recreate Girls) is a health and fitness organization in more than 100 college campuses, empowering women to tackle new health challenges in groups. Members take different classes, such as kickboxing, Pilates, and cardio dance, but it's not just about working out. It's also a way to form a larger, encouraging group and to build a sense of commu-nity. Having friends and feeling good? Yes, please! Fitness clubs and student organizations can be great for accountability. If you've got friends texting you because you're late to a group run, you might be more inclined to show up rather than heading back to bed.

Off-Campus Resources

You can also find local events in the surrounding area. You might find a group that meets at a local park for weekly yoga or a 10K race to put on the calendar as a goal. Is there a local golf course offering discounted memberships? Are there basketball courts with a local meet-up for a young adult season? Kickball? Depending on the environment surrounding your college, see what equipment is available for you to check out to help you explore it. For example, if you're located close to a body of water, you might be able to rent kayaks or paddle boards. If you're in an urban environment, maybe you could rent a bike and explore the city while getting in some endurance exercise. College doesn't stop at the edge of campus, so take advantage of what's around you! Here are some ways to find affordable options.

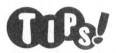

- Check out free, locally sponsored fitness activities. You can usually find ads for these at your local library, community center, town hall, or on flyers around town.

- Do online searches for community, pay as you wish, or sliding-scale pricing facilities. These pay models are based on your income and enable people to participate in an equitable way.

- Always ask about age- or student-based discounts.

- Take advantage of free trials or special promotions.

Self-Led Exercise

Downloadable workout routines are often free and available right to your phone. Search YouTube videos for particular exercises tailored towards your level of fitness and even dorm friendly workouts accommodating for small spaces or living in multi-floored buildings. These at-home and on-demand routines are great for those days when the university gym is overcrowded or when a delayed study session has caused you to miss your normal group workout. If the weather is horrible, or you just don't feel like walking across campus, search for bodyweight routines online where you can get a workout anytime and anywhere. One of the best parts about using an app or a video is that you can search just about anything and tailor a workout to meet your lifestyle and needs. So if you're particularly crammed on time but need a little stress relief, you can crank out a 20 minute workout and get your mind off things for at least a little bit. Save the videos that you enjoy and try free trials on apps before purchasing.

Exercise

Creating Goals and Routines

Once you've found your preferred activity and what resources are available to you, it's time to nail down the last pieces, namely motivation and consistency. That means building a routine and creating realistic goals to keep you motivated. Goals can be small, like adding one exercise routine a week, or large, like training for a marathon. Maybe you already have a routine, maybe you are completely new at this. Here are a few tips to get you moving, literally.

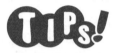

- Don't overwhelm yourself with too much too soon or by taking something too challenging. Start small to build a sustainable habit!

- Listen to your body. If you're not feeling well, skip the workout and catch up on your sleep.

- Keep a journal or have an exercise buddy you can talk to about how you feel after your workouts and what is and isn't working.

- Be kind to yourself. Setbacks are not failure, just an opportunity to grow!

- Identify one area in which you'd like to grow, whether that's building strength, adding in movement, or training for something big.

- Start small to build a sustainable habit!

Outline Your Routine

Activity

Identify Your Goal:

_____

Weekday	Did you Exercise (Y/N)?	Type of Exercise	How Long?	Jot down how you feel afterwards
Monday				
Tuesday				
Wednesday				
Thursday				
Friday				
Saturday				
Sunday				

Priorities for the Weeks

1. _____

2. _____

3. _____

Note, it's important to notice how you _feel_ when you are active and to listen to your body. It takes time to develop a habit, so you'll have plenty of chances to find activities you like the most. In a few weeks, circle back and see what unhealthy stress management skills (like excessive drinking) you've replaced! And if your GPA gets a bump in points, well, that's just an added bonus, isn't it?

Exercise

REFLECTION

What new exercises have you tried? Identify what category of physical activity they fall under. Comment on any overall health and wellness improvements you've noticed thus far.

_____

_____

_____

Write about your first experience using an on-campus, off-campus, or at-home workout facility. Explain how you felt trying something new and possibly out of your comfort zone. Take note of what you liked and didn't like.

_____

_____

_____

_____

What helps you stick to your comprehensive workout routine (from types of exercise to getting enough sleep)? List at least three things.

_____

_____

_____

_____

CHAPTER 5

Nutrition

This chapter will give you some easy starting points for healthy eating, and help you build a sustained balanced diet, even in a college cafeteria. You'll be able to see how eating well can have a major impact on your academics, and your ability to have enough energy to tackle the day. (You'll also see that healthy habits don't mean that you can't still indulge your sweet tooth.) But you will be able to retain a healthy relationship with food even while stressed and you will grow confident in your ability to find balance and consistency in eating well.

It's 11:00 P.M. on a Wednesday night, and you've been cramming for two exams scheduled on Thursday. You once hated coffee, but at the moment it's your only friend, so you grab a cup, and another, and another, as you try to stay up memorizing a few more concepts. You're hungry now, too, but the dining hall is closed, which leaves you with the unappealing options of boiling a cup of noodles, ordering some fast food, or hitting up whatever's in the nearest vending machine. It's not your first all-nighter. You sigh, resignedly cracking open your books, and you don't see it being your last.

This time, it's 11:00 A.M. on a Saturday, you're on a well-deserved hang with your friends, and they're looking to hit up the greasiest burger joint for lunch. Lunch turns into a full day, and as you head into the evening gearing up for a fun night, you all order pizza. You wake up the next morning. It's late, but you're exhausted, so you close the blinds, vowing to yourself that you'll crank out your research paper that's due Monday later in the night, and you hit snooze.

The choices made in these situations feel completely necessary and justifiable in the moment, but they've left you feeling increasingly sluggish and tired. You're not enjoying your classes as much—even hanging out with friends is starting to feel like a chore.

Introduction

Many students find it difficult to establish healthy eating habits in their first year of college (and even beyond). There's a reason why colleges have a reputation for the so-called "Freshman 15," the not so affectionate nickname given to the 15 pounds first-year students tend to gain. There are countless good reasons why this happens—you're already acclimating to a lot of new experiences and responsibilities, and maintaining healthy eating habits might not be at the top of your list—but that doesn't mean it has to happen to *you*, and it's never too late to course-correct, especially if you're not feeling your best.

Consider, for instance, how easy it is to overindulge, especially when you've got a pre-loaded meal card and you don't have a sibling or family member around to call you out on a bad habit. What this means is that if you're righteously using the cafeteria's ice cream machine to unwind, *you* are the one who has to set limits and find balance. The truth is, most students don't eat the recommended serving of fruits and vegetables in a day. This can have an impact on your overall health and, accordingly, how you perform academically. Poor nutrition can result in a lack of focus, affect your cognition and concentration, bring about post-sugar-high crashes, and even lead to larger health issues.

% of college students who reported:	Male	Female	Total
Drinking 0 sugar-sweetened beverages (per day), on average, in the last 7 days	34.6	32.9	33.4
Drinking 1 or more sugar-sweetened beverages (per day), on average, in the last 7 days	65.4	67.1	66.6
Drinking energy drinks or shots on 0 of the past 30 days	73.3	83.3	80.2
Drinking energy drinks or shots on 1–4 of the past 30 days	16.6	11.1	12.7
Drinking energy drinks or shots on 5 or more of the past 30 days	10.1	5.6	7.1

% of college students who reported:	Male	Female	Total
Eating 3 or more servings of fruits (per day), on average, in the last 7 days	17.9	18.4	18.3
Eating 3 or more servings of vegetables (per day), on average, in the last 7 days	29.9	30.8	30.7

Source: American College Health Association—National College Health Assessment, Spring 2020.

This means that the types of food and quality of nutrition available on your campus are important, and what you eat on a daily basis can have a lasting effect. If you have food preferences or health conditions like allergies or diabetes, you have likely already made some adjustments to on-campus dining.

Your college years are some of the most formative years of your life, and there's no better time to build healthy nutritional practices. After all, you're already learning everything, from what values are important to you to how to apply for a credit card; this is simply another skill that will make you happier and healthier during and beyond your college years.

Establishing Healthy Habits

Relatively simple changes in diet can make a big, stress-relieving difference. Even something as simple as eating breakfast can have a positive effect on your GPA because of the effect it can have on your cognitive skills and ability to function. This means that it's important to take lasting steps; we're not just talking about one day of eating healthily, and we're not suggesting that you ditch so-called junk foods and sweets entirely. We are talking about building consistent and nutritious eating habits that will literally fuel your body to be able to handle crunch time for finals, or any other stressors in your life.

Students report that the main barriers standing in the way of healthy eating choices are time constraints, stress, unhealthy snacking, and the availability of junk food. Have you ever found yourself in a similar situation? Check out the following tips to help you plan ahead and prioritize your health:

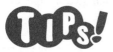

■ Identify where nourishing foods are available on campus. Note even the places beyond the dining hall or a market, like a café hidden at the bottom of your academic building, from which you can grab a quick bite as you run from class to class.

■ Stock up on healthier snacks you prefer from the cafeteria and carry them with you. Keeping a preportioned snack handy will help you avoid overindulging.

■ Prep meals when you have time so that you've got something to eat later when you don't, like if you'll be stuck in a group project or a rehearsal that would keep you from the dining hall.

■ Fill up your water bottle and carry it around with you wherever you go. Drinking a solid amount of water can keep you energized and feeling full.

■ Pay attention to the meals that get your energy going and prioritize time for them in your schedule. If you know breakfast helps you get through the day but you have an early class, note which food places will be open before that time, set an alarm, and get your good eats.

■ Balance your intake of sweet, fatty, and processed foods. You don't have to go cold turkey, but you should be aware of what you're eating and gradually broaden your intake.

■ If you have any allergies or dietary restrictions, speak up and ask if you're unsure about a meal option.

> I found that neglecting to eat well really affected how I did in my classes/extracurriculars because I would get exhausted more frequently and rapidly. Even taking the time to make sure I eat little healthy snacks here and there (yogurt, granola bars, fruits) gave me enough energy to complete my daily tasks.
>
> —*Julia, Williams College*

Access to Nutrition

All of the healthy habits in the world won't make a difference if you can't actually *get* healthy food. Let's look at some of the common places both on- and off-campus, where you can shake things up in a healthy way. We'll also give you some tips and strategies if you don't have easy access to healthy food. Know what's available and get creative, all with the goal of upping your nutrition game.

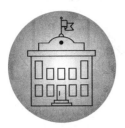

COLLEGE SPOTLIGHT
At the University of California, Berkeley, students can access live virtual cooking classes and nutrition videos put on by Bears in the Kitchen. Students get a recipe and grocery list ahead of time that can be picked up at various locations throughout campus and can then follow along to learn recipes across a wide variety of cuisines.

On-Campus Options

On pretty much any campus, you'll find multiple food sources, whether that's a cafe, a dining hall, or a vending machine. Some are only open during specific hours, so it's good to know what's around you and what's open whether you've just left a late-night study session or an early morning workout and are in desperate need of some fuel.

Breakfast, Lunch, and Dinner

Dining halls, cafeterias, and food courts are your three-meal-a-day staples. They are located throughout campus and are the spots where you can incorporate regular meals into your daily routine. You can use your meal card, get to know your favorite dining options, and sit down for a meal. You might have a cafeteria attached to your dorm and be able to wake up in time to have breakfast before class. You might find a really good station that serves up veggie bowls or salads that will last a few days in a mini-fridge. Keep an eye out for limited offerings, like a customized omelet bar that's only available between 9:00 A.M. and 11:00 A.M.

In larger dining halls, seek out labels that can help you navigate food choices. You might find a color-coded system that defines vegetarian, gluten-free, or plant-based foods. Consider things like convenience, hours of operation, and times where certain food stations are open so you can choose where to eat. Take note of the cafeterias that serve the foods you like and the ones that are offering accessible options tailored towards your allergies and preferences.

COLLEGE SPOTLIGHT

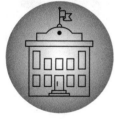

The Florence and Chafetz Hillel House at Boston University provides kosher options for every meal and also offers grab to-go options, all while being included in their meal plan. The main dining hall also offers meals on religious holidays. Check out whether your university has a similar organization at https://www.hillel.org/ and ask dining halls if they provide any options to match your diet. If you don't have access to specific meals, consider local food sources, or even get active with a student group on campus to advocate for more campus amenities.

Late Night and Snacks

Not every schedule fits around the same meal hours, so make sure you know where you can pick up food when the dining hall is closed. Smaller markets and to-go places are convenient places to pick up baskets of fruit, packs of nuts, granola bars, and other quick options. However, they also tend to be well-stocked with goodies like ice cream, chips, energy drinks, and many other products that you may find yourself craving at 10:00 P.M. after a late study session. Know what you are walking into so that you don't exhaustedly grab the first thing you see, especially if it's something that will only drain you further.

The same rule of thumb goes for vending machines, which are open all day! That said, while these are helpful should you lose track of time and need to grab something close to your current location so that you don't lose your spot, there are two things to watch out for. First, know which ones are stocked with healthier, more substantial snacks. Second, be aware of how much they cost, especially if they're not covered by your meal card.

Snacks

List two of your favorite healthy snacks:

1. _____   2. _____

List two of your favorite indulgent snacks:

1. _____   2. _____

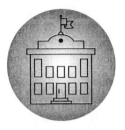

COLLEGE SPOTLIGHT

The University of Arizona and the University of Oregon are two of many universities that conveniently provide to-go smoothies, acai bowls, and other gluten-free, vegan options conveniently housed within their recreation centers so you can work out and take healthy food with you when you go. Other quicker food places might be in areas throughout campus you didn't even think of, like, for example, at the bottom of academic buildings, off the library, or even in the recreation centers and gyms. Ask around, or check online, and make note of places that offer more variety in a pinch.

Stockpiling and Your Dorm

If you have access to a mini-fridge or are buying food that doesn't need to be refrigerated, remember that you can always take your food to go. This is especially useful if you know you're going to have to miss a meal later that day, like if you're going to be busy volunteering during lunch. It's also critical for those students who may need access to foods at all hours. For instance, if you need something like juice at the ready to keep your blood sugar levels raised, keep a stash in your room and carry a bottle around with you. Keep a handy list of those places with healthy, easily transportable options—like a deli counter that can provide you with sandwiches—so that you're always good to go. Here are some more tips for storing food in your dorm:

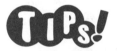

- Save recipes you can make with limited equipment and only a few ingredients to make meals in your dorm so you aren't always relying on outside food sources.

- Have a few ingredients that won't go bad quickly and that will store easily for a meal.

- Have back up snacks stored so if you're running late you can still have an option to grab something before class.

- Check in with your roommate, if you have similar preferences, pool your resources to stay stocked up on snacks and storage spaces, as well as for any appliances your dorm allows, like rice cookers, microwaves, and coffee machines.

- Host a cooking challenge in your hall. A few burnt avocado toasts later, you may find yourself with some terrific makeshift recipes.

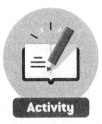

"Home" Cooking

Activity

The convenience of having meals prepped for you cannot be overstated, but, that said, the surest way to have a healthier meal is to control exactly what you put into it. If you don't know how to cook, practice a few simple recipes, ask your roommates, or call a family member for one of their favorite meals. See if your university has cooking lessons, or access videos online to learn everything from how to boil an egg to making homemade lasagna. We've listed a few quick and easy recipes below. Look online for more and then try prepping the ones that seem most appealing or are the easiest to manage. You may surprise yourself.

Recipe

1. **OVERNIGHT OATS**
   Get a jar, fill it with oats, your choice of milk, add some fruit, throw in some chia seeds, stick it in your mini fridge, and in the morning you have a to-go breakfast.

☆ ☆ ☆ ☆ ☆

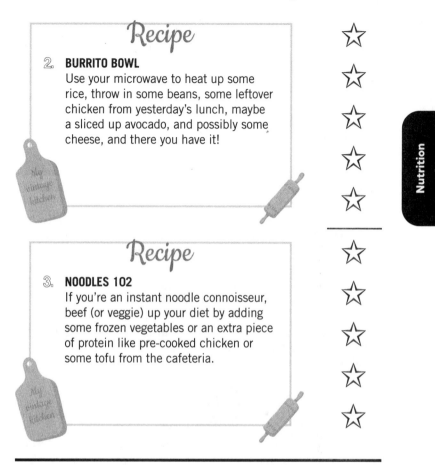

Recipe

2. **BURRITO BOWL**
   Use your microwave to heat up some rice, throw in some beans, some leftover chicken from yesterday's lunch, maybe a sliced up avocado, and possibly some cheese, and there you have it!

☆ ☆ ☆ ☆ ☆

Recipe

3. **NOODLES 102**
   If you're an instant noodle connoisseur, beef (or veggie) up your diet by adding some frozen vegetables or an extra piece of protein like pre-cooked chicken or some tofu from the cafeteria.

☆ ☆ ☆ ☆ ☆

A Note on Food Insecurity

A survey conducted with 3,800 students across colleges and universities, found that 48% of students struggle with food insecurity, which is a lack either of enough food or of access to nutritious and affordable food. This can often lead to students missing classes and study sessions, being unfocused on their academics, having to do without expensive textbooks, and opting out of extracurriculars. On-campus food pantries can be helpful, especially when you eliminate the need to drive off campus to a community food pantry. Colleges may offer free and reduced meals, or alternative meal plans to better fit your needs. If you're struggling with food insecurity, reach out to your university, start with a trusted advisor, or check in with the health center.

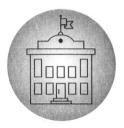

COLLEGE SPOTLIGHT

In March 2021, the Volunteer Center of Butler University opened a food pantry on campus for students in need of food assistance. Students can receive one package per week and place orders in advance, indicating their desired pick-up time, box size, and dietary needs.

Off-Campus Options

Depending on where your campus is located, the surrounding community may be a great resource for finding food. Don't limit yourself to what's closest, either. Once you figure out what's in the area, start to determine how to get there, and maybe even make it into a social event, heading out with a group of friends on bi-weekly or monthly trips to seek fresh provisions. The wider the range of foods available to you, and that may even include ordering from delivery services, the easier it will be to choose healthier options. If you're living off-campus and have access to a kitchen, here are some tips to try:

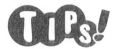

- Don't feel pressured to cook just because you can. This is especially true if you have a mandatory meal plan. Don't forget to use those points when you're on campus, ideally on healthy options.

- Reduce the number of times you have to cook by making larger portions, which you can then store and reheat as necessary throughout the rest of the week.

- Plan to cook or meal prep during downtime. The goal is to make sure you have options even when you're unexpectedly busy.

- Keep a grocery list on hand so that you can restock as efficiently as possible in a single trip.

Nutrition

- Remember that fresh foods will spoil, so try to prioritize cooking these so they don't go to waste.

- If you have roommates, divvy up cooking duties so that you don't have to spend all of your free time prepping. Alternatively, cook *with* friends so you finish faster and have more fun doing it.

Markets and Convenience Stores

Check the local area. If you're in a city and have access to multiple markets and grocery stores, assess which ones fit your budget and your food needs. You might find a smaller market that caters to specific cuisines and that offers ingredients not stocked by larger retailers. You might find a grocery store that has discounts for local students or that offers a rewards program. If you're in a smaller town with fewer options, you should still check what's available, and if you can't find what you are looking for, consider using online retailers to supplement what's available.

Locally Sourced Food

Leaving campus can also be useful for those who want only locally sourced products or more sustainably grown foods. In addition to weekly farmer's markets, you might also find farms that sell fresh eggs, fruits, and vegetables directly to those willing to travel to their property. (These may not be as far away as you think, either!) Of course, some campuses strike up similar deals with neighboring farms, and if they do, you don't even have to travel.

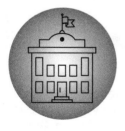

COLLEGE SPOTLIGHT

Loyola Marymount University sources seasonal food from local farms and sources and even has a certification for verified sustainable seafood, tracing what they serve back to the ocean and the docks. The University of Maryland and Portland State University host farmer's markets weekly directly on campus for fresh foods and treats.

Maintaining Healthy Eating Habits

Because you'll be taking different classes each semester, likely with different schedules, you'll need to make sure that your nutritional planning is flexible to accommodate these changes. If you sign up for an extracurricular that will have you in late-night rehearsals, radio broadcasts, or newspaper editing, make sure that you know how you'll get the nutrition you need. It's okay to get off track a bit and it's okay to try new routines, especially as you start a new year or routine. By tracking the things that don't work along with those that do, you can sustain good habits and avoid bad ones and figure out what works best for you as you grow and adapt to new changes, schedules, and challenges. But it is important to pay attention to how you feel and how it affects you day-to-day, so that over time, you feel confident in your own eating habits.

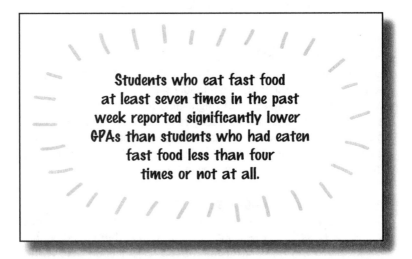

Students who eat fast food at least seven times in the past week reported significantly lower GPAs than students who had eaten fast food less than four times or not at all.

Motivation

There is no greater motivator than *you*. If you're resistant or skeptical about changing your diet, you will sabotage yourself at every turn. Therefore, before you start altering your routine, make sure you know specifically why you're doing it, and give yourself clear and achievable goals to aim for—a week, a month, a semester.

Don't generalize or do something because others—like us—have suggested you should. Get specific and personal. List the ways in which eating well will directly help you. We tend to be more inclined to show up for ourselves when something bigger is at stake, like improving your grades by eating better, especially if those grades will help you get a scholarship opportunity. Let that fuel your decision to, say, start packing healthy snacks as an alternative to candy bars from the vending machine. Some additional motivators can be to:

- have more energy throughout the day

- improve your focus and concentration

- have more time during the day for studies and friends by meal prepping

- maintain a healthy weight

- prioritize a specific diet

- save money by packing snacks throughout the day

- share meals with friends

- get better at cooking

Your reasons for eating healthy might change, and that's okay! You might have moved out from your dorm and now have access to a full kitchen, which then leads you to wanting to cook more meals at home. You might find your dining halls have limited options, and your goal is to find a local or online food service that both caters to your needs and is on a friendly budget. As you go through the school year, assess your commitments, what's available to you, and check your routine to see how you're progressing. Write your goals down, put them in a place where you can see them daily, maybe on a post-it on a mirror, or on the background of your computer, your phone, or wherever you need to place it as a reminder that you're doing positive things daily for a larger reason.

> Creating a routine for yourself is so important. Once you have a routine you'll find that you actually have enough time to do everything you need to do. Exercising and eating well has become a part of my routine and it makes me feel more put together and confident, which honestly translates well into feeling good in class and working with others on big projects.
>
> —*Kimia, University of California, Los Angeles*

Balance

A big part of maintaining healthy eating habits comes from being able to add goodies in moderation. There will be times where you throw your meal plan out the window, or completely walk past the healthy option straight for the frozen yogurt machine. That is okay! Be kind to yourself as you navigate a new environment. Taking one day off is not going to suddenly cause your grades to plummet; in some cases, it might actually reduce your stress. The key is to make sure that these choices are deliberate and not habitual—you're adding in foods you love and enjoy, knowing it's not overindulging to the point where you feel it's too much. In that context, it will be easier to go back to the healthier habits you're trying to establish.

Guidance

Nutrition comes from food, but also from mindset and education, so be sure to get the most out of all the resources your college offers. If you have access to a nutritionist in your recreation or fitness center, try to schedule a consultation. Depending on your campus, you may even be able to get a few free appointments with a registered professional who can speak to your individual needs. The advice you find on the internet and which you get from your friends is likely well-intentioned, but because each student is different, nothing beats a personalized approach, especially if you have food sensitivities or a health history. Dietitians can help you with things like:

- Evaluation of your current nutrition
- Meal planning

- Strategies to introduce and maintain appropriate dietary changes

- General well-being and healthy habits

- Specific dietary needs

- Specific plans for athletes

- Preventing or managing chronic diseases such as high blood pressure, or diabetes

Check academic departments or majors geared towards health and nutrition for additional free services. Even if you're not an athlete, there may be health professionals that are open to working with the general student population. If a nutritionist is not available on your campus, or the price for one-on-one consulting is out of your budget, check for free downloadable apps or campus-wide programming.

COLLEGE SPOTLIGHT

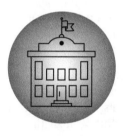

At the University of Texas, Austin students can join a text message service called HealthyhornsTXT and receive texts about campus events, nutrition tips, stress management, and general encouragement to maintain healthy habits. Northern Arizona University has an app where students can see nutrition information, menus, dining hours, and also sync the app with other fitness apps to keep track of daily food intake and create personal goals all from their phone.

Create a Healthy Eating Game Plan

Think of the menu below as a personal tasting menu. Visit as many locations on campus as you can for each meal of the day. You don't have to actually eat at any of these places if you don't see anything appealing, but you will want to make a note of which ones you've ruled out. Be aware of any special properties a dining area has, like if it's the only cafeteria with vegan options, or if it has the only vending machine with healthy snacks. Once you've filled this list, you can go back through and rank your favorite establishments so that you always know where to go, regardless of the hour, for sustenance. The more you write down, the easier it will be to find a back-up if your plans change. (And yes, you can include your own living quarters if you plan on cooking your own meals.)

Depending on the location, the menu may change from day to day. In this case, you may want to visit more than once and if there's a pattern, jot down your favorite, most filling meals so that you don't miss the ones that will leave you feeling healthier, satisfied, and energized. (For places with a fixed menu, this will be easier.)

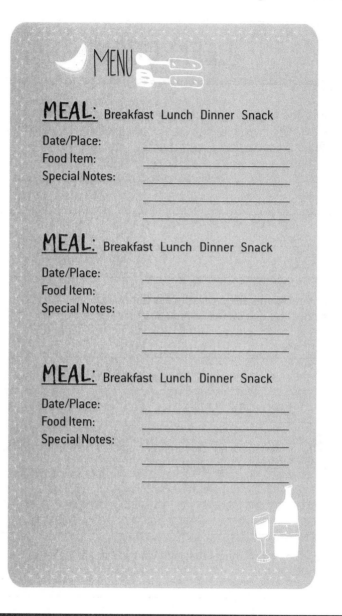

MENU

MEAL: Breakfast Lunch Dinner Snack

Date/Place: _____
Food Item: _____
Special Notes: _____
_____
_____

MEAL: Breakfast Lunch Dinner Snack

Date/Place: _____
Food Item: _____
Special Notes: _____
_____
_____

MEAL: Breakfast Lunch Dinner Snack

Date/Place: _____
Food Item: _____
Special Notes: _____
_____
_____

Nutrition

REFLECTION

What is one way you have incorporated healthier nutrition into your daily routine? How long have you done this for? How does it make you feel?

_____

_____

_____

_____

How comfortable are you with your dining options? What places or ways have you discovered to enhance those options?

_____

_____

_____

How have you used an on-campus resource to help maintain or establish healthy eating habits?

_____

_____

Name at least two things that motivate you to eat well.

_____

_____

_____

CHAPTER 6

Self-Care

This chapter is all about you. You'll learn about the value of self-care, what it entails, and how to incorporate the most effective forms of it into your routine. We'll also look at ways to restore yourself through meditation and sleep, so your body and mind can be recharged for whatever you have going on. By the end of this chapter, you should be well on your way to incorporating mind-clearing activities, better sleeping habits, and other stress-relieving, joy-producing healthy daily practices into your life.

You just got off the phone with your mom. It's only January and she's already asking about grades and your summer plans. You've been thinking about studying abroad, but you have to check with financial aid and your advisor to figure out logistics, and your mind is now thinking about the millions of options, even though summer is months away. You're drained from the conversation and you try to get some sleep, but your thoughts keep you wide awake and overwhelmed.

You were studying fairly late, then your friends texted you to go out to a party. It's been a *week*, and you're really over the books, so you head out. You deserve this. You blow off a few commitments the next day and figure you'll handle it all come Sunday night, maybe even Monday—after all, your exam isn't until Tuesday late afternoon. You push everything back, but then the lack of sleep hits you on Sunday, so you push it back again. The weekend blurs into Monday, and you're just lying there hitting that snooze button. Maybe tomorrow.

It seems like every situation lately leaves you feeling a bit helpless. Your schedule is packed with little room to adjust it, and it feels like you've lost control. Your calendar is the boss. Every day feels the same, and you're trying to get ahead, but you end up rewriting to-do lists, barely finishing assignments, and wanting to ditch your responsibilities altogether. When you're in class, you're thinking about the next commitment; when you're in your club meetings, you're thinking about class; when you're with a friend, you're thinking about how much time you have until your next activity. Finally you get back to your dorm, drop all your stuff, and look at your to-do list. It's like you've hardly made a dent into your tasks.

Introduction

Self-care: it's that small thing you do for yourself that brings a little more joy and ease in your life. It's putting your phone on airplane mode and binging your favorite show uninterrupted. It's taking a long walk and listening to your favorite podcast. It's quality time with a friend. It's any activity that you do to clear your mind and care for your physical, mental, and emotional well-being. It has the power to build resiliency and help you cope with challenges that come your way, and it can simply be a moment in the day where you allow your mind to reframe, refocus, and relax. You have *a lot* on your plate. Whether it's keeping up with classes, squeezing in some time for friends, or remembering to call home and check in with your family even though you're swamped, on any given day there's not enough time and a million tasks on your to-do list.

One of the hardest aspects about self-care is that it can seem so minor in comparison to everything else going on. When you have a research paper, you're running between classes, and trying to connect with friends the last thing on your mind may be to stop and take time for yourself. But the crazy thing about self-care is that, when you incorporate a small practice into your daily routine, you'll actually add more time to your day. Wait, that doesn't make sense, more time? Yes! Because self-care allows you to re-center by giving yourself a little break, which will help you think more clearly and be able to tackle your tasks a bit quicker. Have you ever had those days where you've accomplished a lot, but it feels like you've done nothing? When you're reacting to everything rather than being present in each moment, it can feel like the day flies by, and you've barely caught your breath. This is where self-care comes in. You are allowing yourself to pause for a moment and do something good for yourself, or sit in mindfulness, or even sleep (yes, sleep!). When you do that, you'll reap the benefits. We'll show you how.

If you're feeling stressed about college, take a chance to step back and take a deep breath. Maybe eat or spend time with friends and then come back to whatever you have to do with a fresh mind.

—Emma, Emmerson College

Self-Care

Self-Care

How do you figure out what the right self-care is for you? For starters, self-care will look differently for each person. And what you like might change over time. Allow yourself to try a few different activities and see what works best for you. Here are a few ideas to get you started.

Change Your Scenery

You wake up, grab some breakfast at the dining hall, head to class, head to your next class, grab some lunch, and head back to your dorm. Do it all the next day again. Monotony can be a buzzkill, and it's something we barely notice until a week or two have passed and the days blur together as one. Changing your scenery during the day can do wonders for your energy. Here are some ways to help you switch it up.

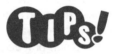

- **Modify your routine.** You have fixed classes to attend and buildings to study in, but if you free up some extra time, you can try taking a different path to get there. Who knows what you'll see along the way?

- **Go somewhere new.** You can either set yourself specific goals, like checking out a museum or a local landmark, or you can choose an area you've never been and explore, whether that's a park or an academic building in which you don't have any classes.

- **Try out different locations.** The dining hall you're eating at might be the most convenient, but is it the best one for your needs? Sure, you've got a great study nook, but might you find an even better one?

Change Your Mood

We know that a long lecture can be a rough way to start the day, and that getting disappointing results back from a quiz or paper can be frustrating. But just as you leave that classroom and move on to the next assignment, shouldn't you similarly try to leave those negative feelings behind? Adding a burst of something you enjoy can help to interrupt and clear up your stress. Here are some ways to change your mood ring to happier color:

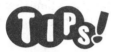

- **Do something for yourself.** If you've been studying all day, find ways to reclaim that activity—read a book for fun, find tutorial videos to watch that are for your favorite hobby, or buy something that's not a school supply.

- **Do something for someone else.** There's no easier way to get out of the problems in your own head than to spend a little time helping someone else with theirs.

- **Entertain yourself.** Music, games, podcasts, television shows—choose something nice to listen to, play, or watch, and you can transport yourself to happier place.

- **Reach out.** If hearing a certain voice brings you comfort, call the friend or family member that you're missing. Even their answering machine might make you smile.

Change Your Pace

It might feel counterproductive to stop working when you're on deadline, but ask yourself how much work you're really getting done when you're exhausted and not thinking clearly. This doesn't just apply to your studying, but to your whole day, especially those that feel unbearably packed. Breaking up your activities and changing your pace can help you regroup and rethink. Here are some suggestions:

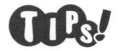

- **Take a timed break.** This isn't an excuse for you to slack off, but rather a way for you to refocus, so give yourself a ten-minute break between assignments as a reward or take a twenty-minute nap to clear your head.

- **Focus on simple pleasures.** Instead of layering task on top of task, do one thing at a time. Set the phone down while you're walking to class or eating a meal and enjoy what you're doing.

- **Change your bedtime.** If you're always feeling rushed in the morning, try going to sleep earlier. If you can't, try sleeping a few minutes less each day until you find the amount of sleep you need. (Note: You may need more sleep, not less!)

Whether it's the scenery, your mood, or your pace, make sure you're changing them for *you*. Contrast any of these with activities that may feel like obligations or which may have consequences, like drinking or partying to an extreme, hanging with someone who drains your energy, or idly scrolling through social media. It's one thing if work or a class doesn't leave you feeling happy and fulfilled (though that's not an ideal situation), but it's another when the things you choose to do for fun also leave you exhausted.

Self-Care of Choice

Write three things you can do for self-care:

1. _____

2. _____

3. _____

Gratitude

You know the expression "Stop and smell the roses?" When's the last time you—with your busy, always-on-the-move schedule—stopped, let alone slowed down? You're at a point in your life that is filled with changes to your environment, commitments, and relationships. You're always striving to accomplish the next thing: You ace one exam, there's another one looming. You make new friends, connect with old ones back at home, only to then study abroad and try to find a new group to connect with while you're away for a few months. You've completed your sophomore year, and now you need to map out junior year. You graduate and now you need to find a job. Take a moment to recognize where you are and what you've accomplished.

Keeping a record of these daily, weekly, monthly, and semester-long successes is an empowering exercise. Each time you stop to appreciate the good things in your life, you're able to refocus on what you can do to get more of them.

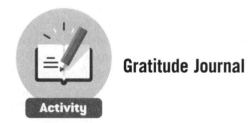

Gratitude Journal

Activity

Open a notes page in your phone in the morning. Write down every good thing that happens to you throughout the day. *If the coffee line was shorter than usual and you make it to class early, write that down! If your friend from home texted you out of the blue to connect, write it down! If you found a 5 dollar bill on the ground, write it down!*

Then, before you head off to bed, write five things you're grateful for and how they make you feel. *Example: I am grateful for my class starting later in the day. I feel at ease knowing I have the morning to get ready, take my time, and sleep if I need to.*

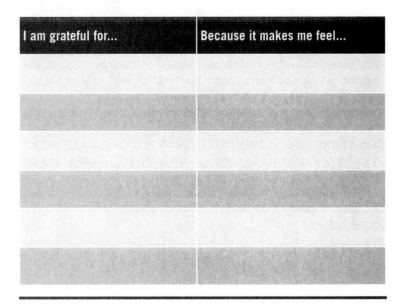

I am grateful for...	Because it makes me feel...

How to Incorporate Self-Care Into Your Routine

By now you have some ideas as to what self-care can look like for you. So how do you ensure it's not just a one-time thing? First, begin by defining some self-care activities you'd like to do. You can refer back to the list from the start of this chapter. Self-care doesn't have to be one thing, and it doesn't have to be complicated. What's important is that it's specifically something you're intentionally doing *for you*.

Next, make sure you've got some regular time for these activities, what some might call "Me Time." Adapt to the schedule you currently have—self-care should never be a burden!—and account for anything joyful you've already scheduled, like performing in a student-run production, or taking part in a regular pick-up flag-football game in your quad. At first, maybe you'll only have ten minutes or so that you can free up—start with that and go from there. Make sure that you internalize self-care by recording or just taking a minute to notice how you *feel* after doing these things. Don't forget about the good parts of your day! It'll keep you motivated to do more and recognize the things you're *already* doing that bring you joy.

Setting Aside "Me Time"

The idea of managing your time may feel a bit like a joke to the average college student. After all, there isn't enough time for everything already on your plate, let alone adding time aside for yourself. But that's the beauty of coming up with a time-management system: the little bit of extra work you put in now will save you a lot of time later, to say nothing of how it adds value to your mental health and alleviates external pressures. So where do you begin?

Look at your schedule for the week and choose a day or two that you have lighter commitments. If you use your phone, set a reminder or a calendar alert ahead of time. If you prefer writing it down, add it with your other commitments and assignments and in a place where you'll see it. Prioritize finding time to sit down and add it to your schedule.

Map out your weekly schedule as carefully as if you were planning a road trip or a vacation. You'll want to have two tiers to your schedule, one that accounts for daily tasks and one that tracks your larger goals. Your day-to-day calendar will have your regular assignments, classes and appointments, and space for extra notes and yes, your self-care and me time. Your monthly planner will look at overall needs—for instance, in August you might want to map out your larger assignments for the whole term by reviewing the syllabi and also making note of any breaks or trips lined up. If it's November, you'll add Thanksgiving break and finals schedules so you can account for time off, travel, and make any weekly adjustments.

There's no set way to track these dates, so long as your method reliably works for you. Many students use digital apps that have built-in reminders, while others prefer dry-erase boards, pocket journals, or post-it notes.

Self-Care

Rethinking the "To Do" List

To be clear, a to-do list is a terrific way to help prioritize a number of things that you have to accomplish throughout the day. But these little lists can become time monsters, with seemingly endless tasks that devour your freedom: finishing class assignments, paying bills, checking in with friends, showing up to that doctor's appointment, it goes on and on. Try reframing your approach by instead calling it a "priority list" or a "success list." If you can't do it all, you can at least celebrate what you've accomplished, and take comfort in knowing that, if you organized the list by importance, you took care of the most critical tasks.

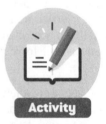

Lighten Your Load

Activity

In each of the balloons below, jot down all the tasks you have to accomplish today. (You can also do this by listing all the tasks you have due this week.) Draw arrows pointing UP or DOWN for each balloon depending on how you answer each of the following questions.

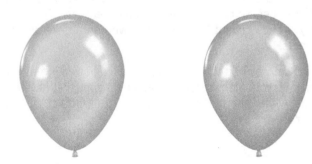

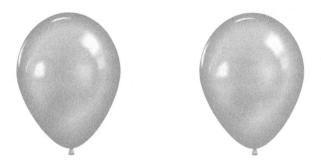

- Move DOWN if you believe the task will be EASY and UP if you think the task will be HARD.

- Move DOWN if you think the task will take LESS THAN AN HOUR and UP if you think the task will take MORE THAN AN HOUR.

- Move DOWN if you can DO THIS ASSIGNMENT ANYWHERE and UP if THIS TASK WILL REQUIRE ADDITIONAL RESOURCES.

- Move DOWN if you feel CONFIDENT about this task and UP if thinking about it makes you OVERWHELMED.

The tasks with the most UP arrows are those that should be your priority!

Self-Care

Meditation

For a lot of students, meditation can feel new and a bit strange. Don't worry, we'll help you out. We have a lot on our minds and it can be difficult to focus and mentally recharge. That's where meditation comes in. Meditation is a practice of attention and awareness, allowing you to observe thoughts without judgment, and gain a sense of calm and clarity. It can help you increase your focus and creativity, and it can also reduce and manage stress and depression. Meditation lets you pause for a moment and breathe, allowing thoughts to come and go and bringing awareness rather than stress to your day.

How do you get started? Meditation can be as simple as closing your eyes and breathing, taking a yoga class, or listening to a meditation app on your phone. It can also be sitting somewhere uninterrupted and listening to your favorite music.

Here's are some tips for getting started:

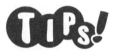

■ **Get comfortable.** Whether you're sitting on the floor, on a mat, or in a chair with your feet firmly planted on the ground, you should be relaxed. (This also means that there shouldn't be any loud noises.)

■ **Be intentional.** Take deep, controlled breaths as you inhale and exhale. Counting as you do so might help you to maintain a regular rhythm.

- **Close your eyes, not your mind.** It's normal for your mind to wander, especially as you start. Just follow your thoughts without judgment as they drift in and out.

- **Set limits, not expectations.** Start by timing yourself for a couple of minutes and just track how your body feels. Starting any new routine will feel different—that's the point—so give yourself time to adjust.

- **Stay consistent.** As you're starting out, don't keep changing your posture, your location, or the time of day, as that can make it difficult to see any difference in your mood.

On-Campus Resources

Check around campus for dedicated meditation spaces. At Hamilton College, there's a space specifically set aside for weekly yoga and group meditation, and it remains open 24 hours a day for any individuals who might need a quiet place to decompress. Other colleges have their own variations on this, like Mount Holyoke College, which has a Japanese Teahouse and meditation garden and the University of the Pacific, which features a reflection pool with benches for students. Find what works best for you whether that's an outdoor space, on a yoga mat in the gym, or at home in your room. See if you prefer music or no music, a guided meditation, or simply a timer for a few minutes in the morning. Notice if you prefer meditation in the morning or at the end of a busy day. There's no one set way to meditate so allow yourself to explore and see what happens! Even if you've never tried mediation before, approach this new practice with an open mind and see what changes. You might be pleasantly surprised with the results!

Downloadable Apps

If your campus doesn't offer classes, or if you want to find a quiet place of your own in which to work independently, consider downloading an app. There are static ones, which take place in a given space, as well as guided walking meditations that can help you find awareness as you move about familiar spaces, breathing in a rhythmic pattern. Most importantly, these programs operate on your time, which makes it a snap to fit them into your schedule. Do be aware, though, that meditation is a routine, so if you set timers and reminders for yourself, you're the only person who can ensure that you're committing to them.

Many apps offer free trials or ad-supported versions, so if you're on a budget or are skeptical of how well this sort of self-directed programming can meet or supplement your needs, you've got nothing to lose in trying them out.

Meditate. Download a meditation app. Go on runs and walks. Eat healthy. It will all work out.

—Isaiah, Syracuse University

The Mindfulness App

This program assesses your current progress and offers you specific ways in which to improve your focus, physical health, or meditation. When you first open the page, the loading screen starts with *Take a Breath*. As you put in your preferences, which include adaptations for beginners, you'll then choose areas you'd like to work on, like getting better sleep, strengthening your physical health, reducing stress, or improving focus. It will recommend a certain number of activities per day based on your preferences and you can set alerts that'll provide you with encouraging messages and reminders to help keep you on track. You can choose courses aimed at your goals, whether that's just learning how to meditate, or focusing on your sleep, and even a travel meditation section for quick exercises you can do on a plane heading back home, on a trip, or anywhere you feel the need! There's a free trial and if you're not wanting to commit to the full year after, you can choose one month to subscribe to a specific topic rather than the entire program.

Headspace

Headspace has a variety of videos, guided meditations, and a *move* section with stress-relieving workouts and stretches. In the focus section, you can find meditations and music playlists, throw on your headphones and turn them on while studying. If your mind is racing right before bed and you're thinking about all the things you need to do, the sleep section has a mental chatter meditation. There's an *SOS* section if you're feeling panicked, anxious, or generally burned out, and with a calm voice you'll be guided as you step away from worried thoughts and help settle your mind.

For the Skeptics

A group of students at the University of Rhode Island underwent a six-week yoga and meditation course in preparation for final exams.

> At the beginning of the study, over a third of the students reported having high stress. By the end of the study, students reported a significant decrease in stress and anxiety. They also reported an increase in feeling aware and mindful.

This isn't rocket science: a person's focus is tied to their awareness and mindfulness, so improving those areas helps to maintain your concentration. In turn, that added focus makes it possible to more easily retain information, analyze situations, and problem-solve. These are all things that will help you in your studies and, of course, ace your finals.

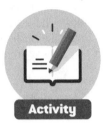

Activity

Five Senses to Destress

This technique can be used whenever you feel overwhelmed, anxious, or stressed. Write down what's stressing you the most right now and go through each sense, keeping track of how you feel throughout.

What's the one thing stressing you out?

_____

_____

👁 Look at **five things** around you. Write them down.

_____

_____

✋ Touch **four things** around you. Write each down.

_____

_____

👂 Listen to **three things** in the area. Write each down.

_____

_____

Smell **two things** in the environment. Write each down.

_____

_____

What **one thing** do you most taste right now? Write it down.

_____

Notice how your attention has shifted, how your body feels, and how present you are in this moment. Use this exercise at any point you feel stressed.

Sleep

If you've ever seen an old-fashioned zombie movie and pulled an all-nighter, you probably know that shambling feeling, where it's about all you can do to put one foot in front of the other. You know you're not performing at your best, and that's because you're not getting enough sleep. When your brain gets all foggy and your body snores with every movement, you need sleep.

In a health survey administered to over 30,000 students by the University of Georgia, 1 in 4 students say that lack of sleep has impacted their academic performance in a negative way, and that pulling all-nighters and cramming last minute can actually be counterproductive.

Self-Care

Just as you recharge your phone or fill your stomach, you need to refuel both your mind and body by giving them a chance to shut down, rest, and conserve energy for the next day. On average, teenagers need eight to ten hours of sleep, and adults over eighteen need seven hours. This is especially important when you have big events coming up, which is why cramming for a test can be so dangerous if it means you then have to *take* the test while you can't focus. So let's look at ways you can get in your Z's.

Go to Bed!

First, we recognize you're in college, so yes, there will be nights where you're out late doing your thing or you're messaging your friend, and it cuts into your sleep. You're human, and you're allowed to have fun. Everything in moderation, right? But in general, creating a consistent sleep schedule and establishing habits to help wind your mind and body down will, hands down, give you better sleep. Why? Because your body will begin to pick up on clues when it's time to go to bed. And the more consistent you are with the time you go to sleep, the time you wake up, and the things you do *before* getting ready for bed, all set off signals it's time for sleep.

Here are some tips to keep your sleep regulated:

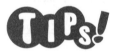

- **Don't oversleep on the weekends.** If you normally wake up at 8:00 in the morning, but regularly sleep until 1:00 in the afternoon on the weekend, it might be time to make a change.

- **Create a routine before bed.** Give your body cues that it's time to wind down. This can be making a cup of tea, journaling, reading, washing your face, brushing your teeth, and having a relatively consistent bedtime.

■ **Set your space up for a serene environment.** Get rid of anything that keeps you up. If the room is too bright, dim or turn off the lights. If your phone keeps buzzing or lighting up, disable that function or put it where the light won't disturb you. If you've got a noisy, uncooperative roommate, get an eye mask, put on your headphones, and listen to some white noise.

■ **Don't study on your bed.** If you're in a dorm, this may not be so easy, but try to make your bed a place for resting, not studying. You want to send clear signals to your body that it's time for sleep, not work.

■ **Exercise.** Although you may feel physically exhausted after exercising, that's not a good time to go to sleep. Give yourself a few hours between any full-body workouts and bed so that your heart rate can come down and your body can switch into recovery mode.

■ **Avoid caffeine.** At the very least, don't drink it within a few hours of bedtime, so that you can let your body metabolize the caffeine before it sleeps.

■ **Have a journal or notebook next to your bed.** Instead of mulling over what you're going to tell someone, write down what you're thinking to get it out of your system so you can sleep.

Sleep Cycles

It's worth mentioning the science of sleep cycles. Don't worry, there won't be a lab on this, unless you count tracking your sleep for the best results. But for the sake of simplicity, you have two basic types of sleep, rapid eye movement (REM) sleep and non-REM sleep, which also has a few different stages. They all connect to your brain activity, and you cycle throughout both REM and non-REM sleep multiple times throughout the night, ultimately landing on a deeper REM period in the morning.

As you settle down in that cozy dorm bed, with extra-long twin fitted sheets no doubt, your heartbeat, breathing and eye movements will all slow down and your muscles will relax. You'll enter a lighter non-REM period and then into a deeper one and end up in that REM cycle toward the morning. Your body also goes through something called circadian rhythms. No, this is not a dance move, but the rhythms direct some functions in your body, including your body's biological clock. Just a fancy way of saying, your body will respond to cues in your surroundings like light and temperature and the time of day that can help trigger you to sleep quicker. So remember that tip of creating consistent surroundings? That'll help promote your body to wind down and also wake up at a consistent time.

Then there's the sleep-wake homeostatic sleep, which reminds the body it needs to sleep and it also regulates how deeply you sleep. Things like medications, stress, what you put in your body, and your environment can all influence your sleep-wake. You know your body best, so it's helpful to pay attention to habits and routines that either help or hinder your sleeping situation.

Naps

Naps can be a beautiful thing. Approximately 30 to 50 percent of college students nap. So more sleep is obviously a good thing, right? Well, not necessarily. Naps can also be a beast if you find yourself frequently napping for solid amounts of time. If you're a nap person or want a bit more energy, the best way to enjoy the benefits is to close your eyes for 10–20 minutes midday or in the early afternoon. Remember those REM and non-REM cycles? If you nap later on into the evening, you're entering the deeper REM stages, which could possibly disrupt your ability to fall asleep. If you're finding yourself needing more energy and a nap just isn't going to cut it, whether that's due to you cutting into sleep time or worrying about napping straight through chem lab, consider taking a walk or just sitting in the sun.

When Your Sleep Becomes a Concern

Just like seeing a doctor for a physical ailment or a counselor for a mental health concern, consulting with a health professional is important if you're finding your sleep is becoming more of an issue.

Here are a few indicators it might be time to get an expert opinion:

- You regularly experience difficulty with sleep

- You fall asleep at inappropriate times, even after a full night of good sleep

- You have night terrors constantly that interrupt your sleep (you wake up in an anxious or fearful state without remember dreaming)

- You have trouble getting through your day without exhaustion

- You fall asleep while driving or frequently in class

- You struggle to stay awake during activities that don't require much energy (like watching TV)

- You have difficulty paying attention or concentrating in school

- You notice lack of sleep affecting your academic performance

- You have memory difficulties

- You have difficulty controlling your emotions

- You need naps daily (and not just the 10–20-minute quick nap we discussed previously)

Self-Care

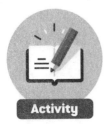

Sleep Tracker

Activity

Instructions: Shade in the portions of each pillow for which you accomplish your sleep task on the right.

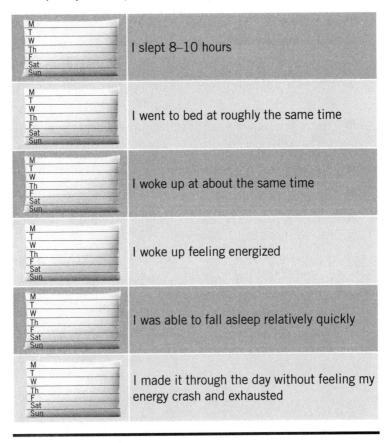

Pillow (M, T, W, Th, F, Sat, Sun)	Sleep task
M T W Th F Sat Sun	I slept 8–10 hours
M T W Th F Sat Sun	I went to bed at roughly the same time
M T W Th F Sat Sun	I woke up at about the same time
M T W Th F Sat Sun	I woke up feeling energized
M T W Th F Sat Sun	I was able to fall asleep relatively quickly
M T W Th F Sat Sun	I made it through the day without feeling my energy crash and exhausted

REFLECTION

What new self-care activities have you tried? Identify which ones you like best and comment on how you felt after, if it relieved some stress, brought you joy, etc.

_____

_____

_____

What's one way you can incorporate self-care into your routine? Whether that's keeping a calendar, setting reminders in your phone, be specific.

_____

_____

Try meditating for at least 2–3 minutes. Remember, this can be just sitting and breathing! Write how you felt.

_____

_____

On average, write how many hours of sleep you're getting per night. What's one thing you can do to improve your sleep (whether that's sleep quality, or increasing the number of hours, or eliminating the snooze button).

_____

_____

Self-Care

CHAPTER 7

Study Support

This chapter is all about studying effectively. We'll discuss the different types of tutoring and how each one can help you in different ways, as well as things like library resources and help from academic departments. We'll give you tips on how to form effective study groups as you learn how to better structure your time and establish healthy group boundaries. Finally, we'll look at how to make the most of your environment, with ways to make any place in your home or campus into a comfortable place to study.

Thanksgiving break is over and final exams are just around the corner. A true procrastinator at heart, you've been accustomed to cranking out assignments in high school, snagging points here and there over the entire semester. This semester, your grade relies largely on a midterm and a final exam, and you're in panic mode. Studying has never been your jam and it seems impossible to review months of material in the little time you have left. It gets harder to suppress the rising anxiety of what December will bring.

It's Wednesday evening, and your first debate in your political science class is tomorrow. This wouldn't have felt so intimidating if it weren't for the size of the class: it's just you, 10 other students, and the professor, and you're worried about being embarrassed when you have to present without notes. While your bedroom door is closed, the party downstairs is very much open and it's too loud to think, so you head to the student union, but you find the chairs uncomfortable, and the space limited to the point where the party noise has just been replaced with student noise. You're annoyed, your brain is going a million miles per hour, and you feel pretty defeated.

You love your friends, but every time they get together for a study session, you feel like you're learning more about the latest buzzy podcast as opposed to reviewing for exams. It's been fun seeing them, but you're not getting any work done, and the last few times you've brought this up, they've brushed off your concerns. You've considered finding a new group that actually wants to study, but you feel obligated to stick with your friends, and now you have to battle not only the feeling of ditching some much-needed studying time, but also the guilt of ditching your friends.

Introduction

Let's face it: there's never going to be enough time on campus to do everything. What it comes down to, in the end, is just finding the most *efficient* way to handle your responsibilities, so that you can cram even more in without overwhelming yourself. That's where it's helpful to put together support for your studies. For instance, there's likely a place in the library filled with texts pertinent to whatever subject you're studying. Instead of starting from scratch each time and looking through online rabbit holes, you can go directly to those library services and communicate with experts who can point you in the right direction, saving you time and stress.

You can find similar relief when it comes to writing your research papers, especially for the tricky stuff like using the proper citations—what's the difference between APA or MLA?—and keeping your thoughts organized so they're not lost in a sea of open tabs on your laptop. Your school likely has some sort of writing center that you can book an appointment with, or at least a variety of tutoring services that you can avail yourself of throughout the year, based on your needs.

In addition to faculty-led services, like review sessions that help to focus on the key concepts you need to know for tests, you can also make better use of your peers by joining study groups. Setting aside a dedicated time on your calendar to work with classmates can be rewarding in of itself, whether it's a temporary time for one critical assignment or a regular session that's building toward a larger goal and keeping everyone on the same page. When you find the right group, it can also be immediately relieving, as you're getting advice and insight directly from those in your same situation: you're not alone when you have numbers on your side.

Finally, don't overlook the self-guided resources found across campus. Knowing which rooms or buildings are the quietest or most comfortable getaways to study in is invaluable, especially if you're still negotiating how to make peace with your roommate. (We've got you covered with tips for that, too!) Figuring out how to access any advanced computer services (like 3D printers) can save a lot of time and energy, too.

Study Support

Once you put all of these components together, studying will feel like more of a creature comfort—a regular, enjoyable part of your routine—as opposed to a chore that keeps you from putting other social events on your calendar.

Types of Support

You're a part of a larger university and with that comes academic support beyond the classroom. These are the extras that will bring your B to an A or a half-finished paper into a full-fledged and appropriately cited paper. Most of these services are free and accessible on a weekly, if not daily, basis. You don't have to do it all on your own!

Graduation levels have been increasing over the last decade, but according to the National Center for Education Statistics, the rate of those graduating within four years is still under 50%, and those graduating within six years is under 70%. If you feel yourself slipping and stressing, these are some of the developing offerings that can help.

Tutoring

The type of tutoring you pursue depends on your needs. It's helpful to know what's offered, especially if it's already embedded in your fees or otherwise free for you to access (most are). Don't get hung up thinking that there's only one type of tutoring and ignore other options because you once tried one-on-one tutoring and you didn't find it helpful. (This is especially true at the college level, where you may also pick up some great general study tips.) There are all kinds beyond the traditional private options, whether in-person or online. There's also drop-in, small-group, and peer tutoring; programming and services through a writing/academic center; and a variety of review sessions.

You'll also want to be on the lookout for differentiated levels of tutoring. At first, you might be looking out for generalized strategies to help adapt to the college workload, or to a specific teacher's methods. As you progress through your major, you may also find specific tutoring options for those higher-level classes, or even for graduate-level exams like the GRE or MCAT.

Drop-in Tutoring

Some students have this notion that tutoring is something you set up months in advance, at the start of a class, and which you continue to use throughout the semester. In doing so, they miss out on the chance to get immediate and specific help should they end up later getting stuck. If you're trying to unpack a new concept, develop and apply a tricky technique taught in class, or get a quick referral about a topic, consider just dropping by your local tutoring center. If your school offers general tutoring and subject-specific tutoring, find the one that's most pertinent to your burning question. We recommend dropping by at least once, even before you need the help, just to familiarize yourself with the location and the process/availability of a potential walk-in session.

PROS

✔ You may be able to get help more immediately, as opposed to having to wait for an appointment.

✔ There tend to be more drop-in options for general and popular courses, and these tutors are likely to be very familiar with what you're struggling with.

✔ Seeing other students waiting for help can help to emphasize that you are not alone, and that asking for assistance is not just normal but expected.

Study Support

Group Tutoring

You don't always have to go it alone, and we don't mean just in the sense of trying to get everything done without a tutor. You can often find small-group tutoring, where instead of it just being *you* trying to get through a course, you're with others who have similar struggles. If you feel uncomfortable airing your concerns around strangers—though it can be beneficial to see and hear how others are struggling, as you might pick up ideas from one another—you can also make an appointment with a group of your own friends.

PROS

✔ Those in your group may ask questions you hadn't yet realized you needed an answer for, or which you don't feel comfortable opening up about.

✔ Discussing a tutor's advice may help you to better adapt it to your routine. This can also open up other ways to supplement one strategy with others.

✔ If those in your group are also in your class, you may be able to work with them to reinforce the use of key techniques.

Writing Centers

Writing centers offer a specific type of tutoring, one that acknowledges the learning curve that students may face in moving from high-school level research papers to the more complex ones required by college professors. (This is especially true when it comes to perfecting portfolio submissions and dissertations.) Note that departments, especially those that have their own stringent policies for papers, may have their own writing centers, so make sure you're reaching out to the right one for your needs. That said, be sure to check out the general writing center as well, because that overall advice can be very useful. For instance, Hamilton College offers all of its students a handy PDF called *The Seven Deadly Sins of Writing*, which can help to avoid a lot of future rewrites and heartache.

PROS

✔ Writing support is often more targeted than standard tutoring. That is, you can submit a draft and get specific feedback for that paper. Just make sure that you're keeping track of the general advice you get so that each session improves your future writing, and not just for that one assignment.

✔ If you send your paper to a tutor with enough advance notice, you can get a more detailed and helpful discussion out of it—the longer your paper, the more lead time you'll want to provide.

✔ The ability to submit multiple drafts can help you to make gradual improvements and also improve your time-management, since if you're using a writing center in this fashion, you won't be able to wait until the last minute to write your paper.

Online

We've all been there—you're in the middle of a great study session and are making a lot of progress, when you suddenly realize that there's something you don't fully understand. You can e-mail the professor or message a classmate, but there's no guarantee when they'll be able to get back to you, and it would waste a lot of time to have to march out to a drop-in session, if any are even available. That's where online offerings can be especially useful, whether that's providing you with a walkthrough or tutorial video or connecting you to someone who can give a quick, immediate answer. For those who prefer distance, you may also be able to schedule normal tutoring sessions online as opposed to in-person, which is a nice convenience to have. Online services also tend to be integrated, as they are at George Washington University, which means that instead of trying to find the right help center, you can just browse by department and class until you find the right set of resources for you.

PROS

- ✔ Most online tutoring will tell you exactly when there's availability, so you're never waiting around. It also tends to be specifically tailored to your question, so you're being matched with someone who knows exactly what information you need.

- ✔ Reaching out to an academic ensures that you're pulling from reputable resources as opposed to third-party sources or blogs that may get you in trouble on a paper.

Digital Toolkit

Name a free online resource your university offers that could be of use to you.

_____

_____

Review Sessions

We know many students are eager to shut down their computers and get out of the classroom as soon as they can, but don't be so hasty. Heading back to class for a bonus review session, whether that's led by the teacher, their assistant, a graduate, or a peer, can be a great way to back up what you've been learning. Don't think this support is only for a particularly tricky subject, either. The more you reinforce your knowledge now, the easier it will be to reconnect to it when you're studying for a test down the road. If your school offers one-time or recurring sessions, give it a try and see how it impacts your retention.

PROS

✔ When universities sponsor these sessions, they tend to hire experienced students to sit through classes so that they can help new enrollees. This means that you're not only getting the expertise from *this* class, but from everything else that student has picked up since they first took it.

✔ These sessions tend to have fewer students in attendance, which gives you the opportunity to ask and unpack questions you've been carrying around since lecture.

✔ Review sessions can help you to provide structure and accountability—it's a lot easier to put off your independent reviewing for another night than it is to skip a pre-test review.

✔ Official sessions may also offer samples from previous tests, which can be a good way to make sure you're prepared for high-stakes midterms or finals.

"Graduate instructors saved my life... [they teach] everything the teacher missed in the lecture. They were helpful in their discussion classes and SO helpful in their office hours. I got an A in numerous classes because of their help."

—*Emily, University of California, Berkeley*

Private Tutoring

The options we've discussed thus far have been largely campus-related, but note that your school may also have partnered with private tutors, and if you need additional support, you should investigate what sort of discounts and offerings are available. There are various platforms and models, ranging from hourly rates to a one-time access fee that's good for a period of time, and signing up in a group (with your friends) can help to further reduce the cost, if there is one. Free trials are also frequently offered, which can give you a sense for how a private tutor differentiates their services from anything school-provided: generally speaking, this tends to be a wider and more personalized range of expertise and services.

PROS

✔ Paid online tutoring, like our own at Tutor.com, tends to be offered 24/7, which can be very helpful in a late-night study session in which you find you need immediate help.

✔ On-campus offerings may be limited in terms of available volunteers, but private tutors or companies provide a wider selection, so you can find not just the help you need but the specific *tutor* that you need.

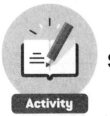

Strategy Guide

All the useful pointers and strategies you receive from tutors, advisors, and your peers won't amount to anything if you don't find ways to regularly implement them into your routines. Use the following worksheet to list strategies in your own words and then account for the places in which you've tried them. If they were unsuccessful, put an X in one of the boxes—fill all three and then determine if you want to keep trying this strategy, or if you want to get rid of it. If you're keeping the strategy, or it was a success, jump down to that final box and think about any new modifications you made or which you want to try out next time, so that this technique is always becoming more useful and more personalized to you.

Strategy Guide

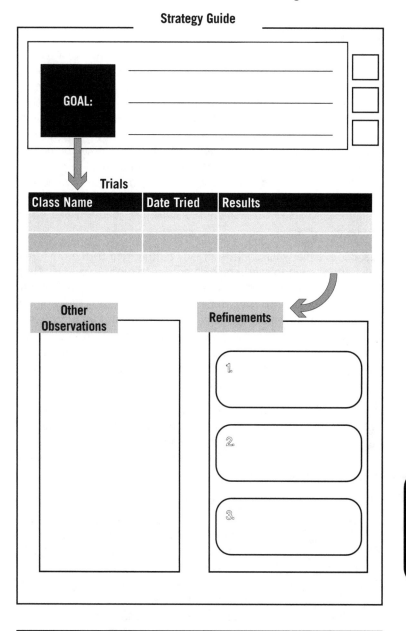

GOAL:

Trials

Class Name	Date Tried	Results

Other Observations

Refinements

1.

2.

3.

Study Support

Library Services

Though a librarian might not teach a specific class that you're taking, there's a lot that you can learn from these faculty members, most of whom hold master's degrees and possess a wide and diverse range of information that's right there for the taking. That's especially useful if you're at a school with a large library that's intimidating to search through, or if your school utilizes a sharing network that might be able to deliver you materials from other branches. Beyond books, many libraries also store dissertations, in case you want to get inspiration from graduates. They may also have access to extensive archives—either in microfiche or now, more commonly, in digital formats—of newspapers, magazines, journals, and other reputable sources.

Chances are that your brain is already a little fried by the time that you start heading to the library, so go directly to the experts. They can either walk you through their database search tool or simply direct you to the material you need. They can also likely make recommendations on additional content you might want to look into for your research. In some cases, you might not even need to go directly to the library to access these resources; some universities provide 24/7 access to library support not just through their own school, but with librarians nationwide.

Think of librarians as informational caddies for your student golfing; sure, you *can* carry all your equipment yourself, and figure out exactly what the best tools for the job are . . . or you can trust these experts to help carry some of the load so that you can focus on getting a metaphorical hole-in-one on your paper.

COLLEGE SPOTLIGHT

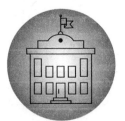

At the University of Puget Sound's Collins Memorial Library, students can book an appointment with a library liaison who is an expert in their respective field. Liaisons provide extensive information on research for particular courses and will provide additional information and strategies when students need help on a topic. Through a competitive hiring process, peer research advisors are employed by the library and available to help their peers in particular subject areas and have a wide knowledge of research tools and strategies.

Study Groups

Peer pressure is often dismissed as negative force that leads to bad behavior, but by the same token, it can also be used for positive reinforcement. The clearest evidence for this is when it comes to the accountability of working on a group project or being part of a study group. When it's just you, there's nothing stopping you from procrastinating or delaying. When others are relying on you to meet up or to contribute work, it's a lot harder to just blow a deadline off. If you're the type of learner who benefits from group settings, make sure you either find—or start—a study group. Diversity is great in these groups, as it means that you're likelier to be exposed to new and useful techniques and discussions; the only thing that you should all be on the same page about from the get-go is your level of dedication to the work. If it helps, think of it a bit like a lower-stakes version of *The Hunger Games*: when your grade is on the line, you want to surround yourself with those who will help protect it.

Formal

A formal study group essentially schedules regular meetings that operate just like class, and you're expected to show up and contribute. These groups tend to be more serious, and can sometimes be run by the school itself, but they're also likely to be driven entirely by the work and may not have as much variety.

Informal

An informal study group can be just as serious as a formal one but may meet less frequently—perhaps only before tests. If you don't have a lot of spare time to dedicate to studying for this class, or don't need that much support, this might be the ideal setting for you. That said, if you're not regularly meeting with your peers, you may not all know the best way to review material or to focus on the work itself.

Whether you're starting your own group or joining someone else's, it's important to be clear about what you're looking for. If there are a few to choose from, maybe try more than one. You may be surprised to find that you learn more in a less serious setting. Alternatively, you may discover that you're more easily confused in a group than when you're on your own, or that any group larger than two or three members makes you feel overwhelmed.

Study Support

Incidentally, as long as the other members are OK with it and you're comfortable with your grades, there's no *wrong* way to conduct a study session. If you're not covering that much material but you *are* getting more comfortable with your classmates, that lessened social anxiety can help you to focus during the test itself. There's ultimately no difference between a study buddy who is distractingly silly and one who is overbearingly erudite if you can't connect with either one. If the group's not a good fit, walk away.

COLLEGE SPOTLIGHT

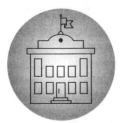

Carnegie Mellon University's Student Academic Success Center offers guidance in helping students form peer-led study groups. Staff will help the group identify their type of study group, whether that's goal oriented (a common mission such as a singular project or exam) or semester-long (an understanding of the overall course material) and from there help students create a schedule that will work for all members. There's even a group agreement helping students establish and maintain boundaries and mission statements and also workshops to help foster more effective study habits as a group.

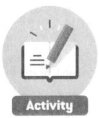

Activity

Creating an Effective Study Group

The best kind of study group is a unified one. For that reason, you want to make sure there's a very clear goal or theme for the group that everyone agrees upon. (This will help to cut down on distractions and disruptions.) In the following box, work out that specific goal—"I want to study better" is way too general—and then break it down with actions you can collectively take to get there. Use the clock icon to break down how much time each session should be and what percentage of each session should be spent on each of those actions, such as reviewing definitions, doing quick quizzes, or collaborating on homework. Incentives can also help with a study group, so at the bottom of this activity, put some sort of group reward—a trip to the movies, a potluck, a pizza party—that will help to keep you focused on your overall growth. You can also set aside some bonus time each session as a break between segments—just mark that on the sheet as well so that you don't end up spending valuable study time on a discussion about the latest reality television breakup.

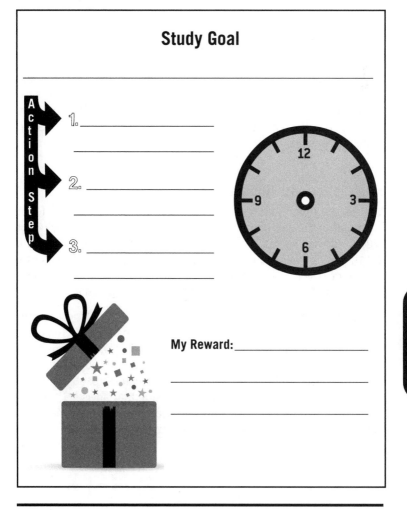

Where to Study

It's probably safe to say that when you attended high school, you had far fewer choices about where to study. While we certainly don't want you to stop using the tips and tricks that have historically worked best for you, we also don't want you to limit yourself from exploring everything now available to you. You may also find that your new circumstances will require you to adapt old surefire techniques to your new digs—for instance, you may have once had your own room, whereas now you'll likely have a roommate or two.

At Home

Even if you don't like studying at home, it's inevitable that the odd hours of college may cause you to have to do some work there. (Maybe that's because your favorite library nook is taken or because the outdoor patio by your favorite restaurant is closed.) Here are a few tips to get you through, regardless of what your home situation actually looks like:

Negotiating with Roommates

You and your roommates will likely have schedules that differ for at least part of the day, and if you know you work best when they're not around (or vice versa), it's a good idea to swap schedules and mark out the times where you'll have the dorm all to yourself. This is true no matter how many roommates you have, and coordinating schedules is a skill that you'll find invaluable once you graduate.

If you still can't get enough private studying time, try to communicate with your roommate about what would help each of you get work done. The earlier you do this in the school year, the more likely you'll both be able to work any necessary concessions into your routine. If you continue to have issues, or can't broach the issue with your roommate, speak with your residential advisor (if you're in a dorm) or try to get a neutral third party—a common friend, or another roommate—to help find common ground.

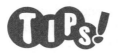

These life-hacks can make it easier to manage a small space or an inconsiderate roommate:

■ **Maintain a dedicated workspace.** Whether you prefer to work on your bed or at a desk, give yourself a consistent, clear area that sends your body the message that it's time for work (as opposed to gaming, or sleeping). The more serious you are about establishing your space, the easier it will be to stay focused.

■ **Turn things around**. Something as small as clearing your desk or rotating it so that it's facing a blank wall as opposed to a window can help you focus.

■ **Tune the outside world out.** Blackout curtains can help you to ignore what time it is outside and noise-cancelling headphones (or earplugs that tune into a free white noise channel) can help to drown out competing thoughts.

■ **Make your distractions disappear.** Stow your electronics by either time-locking unnecessary browsers and applications or putting your phone away.

On Campus

If you don't have enough time to make it back to your room between classes or extracurriculars, or you know there are too many distractions at home, you may be able to find homes away from home on campus. Look for physical spaces that are either already designed for studying—computer labs, empty classrooms—or those that can be repurposed as such, like quiet nooks with comfortable counter spaces and nearby charging stations.

The Library

We spoke about the resources available at the library before from a research perspective, but the generally quiet atmosphere of the library makes it a decent place to work in as well, especially if there

Study Support

are printers, computers, and copiers that you can make use of. Check out the various floors and find the places where it's easiest to read and/or write without interruption.

Classrooms

Depending on your school's policies, some classrooms or library rooms may be available after hours. Do be clear about the hours for these areas, however, because if you're using something specific to that space, like a whiteboard or projector, and get kicked out of the room, you may lose your work. On the whole, these areas are excellent places to hold study group meetings or to rehearse for an oral presentation.

Labs and Studios

Sometimes you need a space that caters to a more specific need than your average classroom space. For instance, if you're experimenting on a design, you might need access to high-end equipment like a 3D printer or might need tools specific for soldering materials together. If you're a performer—a musician, dancer, or actor—you might need a sound-proofed rehearsal room, an artist might need a space to work on a larger-scale project (or to better work with messy components), and a filmmaker might need access to editing software and cameras. These spaces, if available at all, tend to need to be reserved, and will likely go first to those who are majors in that given area, so be sure to coordinate with the right department about their use. That said, professors understand that some students need extra exposure to equipment so as to familiarize themselves with use and reduce anxiety; you definitely can't take advantage of resources if you never ask for them.

Study Lounges

Some dorms and academic spaces have areas where students can study. Some of these are technology focused, so that those who don't have ready access to computers or printers in their dorm can still get their work done in a reliable fashion. Just be aware that while these areas are usually isolated spaces from the rest of the building, they are often communal, which means you'll likely be sharing that space with other students. On the positive side, most students who go to a space like this are in the same boat as you— they're there to study.

Best-Kept Secrets

The campus is largely designed for its students, and unless you're specifically told that an area is off-limits, you should feel free to stake out any nooks and crannies that you discover. Just understand that ownership of these areas is tenuous, by which we mean first-come, first-serve. To that end, it's good to find as many comfortable spots around campus as you can so that you've always got a go-to place in which to do some last-minute studying. Here are some tips:

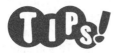

■ Unless you're planning to always study between the same two classes, you should scope out your secret getaway at various points of the day. You may find foot traffic and noise levels to be unbearable at another time.

■ Bring snacks with you. Having your own food and water means that you can scout out areas further away from popular dining locations and snack machines.

■ You aren't restricted from visiting buildings based on your major, and sometimes it can actually be helpful to head to an area that's likely to have fewer familiar distractions.

■ If you're not on deadline, try to fit the work you have to the space you've found. Don't squander that evening's reading assignment in the empty rehearsal room you found if you could instead be working on something that takes up more space. You can do that reading anywhere, like while you're waiting for your laundry to finish drying. Are you comfort-able rehearsing by the washing machines?

■ You can always ask friends for tips, but don't be surprised if they don't share them. After all, you might want to keep some quiet spaces for yourself.

Study Support

The Study Treasure Map

Draw or describe up to three of the spaces that you like to study in on the "treasure" map below and leave some notes for yourself about landmarks that they're near and times that they're most useful to you. You don't have to draw to scale but do try to give yourself a sense of where you're clustering your study sessions. It may be that there are areas yet to be explored, and if one of the areas you've labeled isn't quite up to snuff, you'll know to give the surrounding area another pass. This is about providing yourself with comforting options, not just for this semester, but for your entire college career.

REFLECTION

How have you utilized tutoring to help you in a class? What can you do to get more, if necessary, out of these sessions?

_____

_____

Which type of study group—formal or informal—do you find more appealing? If you have, or plan to start your own, what bad study habits are you hoping to keep out of your group?

_____

_____

Identify at least one area on campus where you study best. What do you find most helpful about this space? How can you incorporate this space into your study routine?

_____

_____

What's one small thing you can incorporate into your daily routine, that will help you with your studying (time management, rearranging your space, etc.)?

_____

_____

Study Support

CHAPTER 8

Community

In this chapter you will learn about places on campus where you can find people who will offer you academic and emotional support and be able to identify who will make up your support system. And don't worry, if the thought of walking around a club fair and going up to booths asking questions seems absolutely terrifying, we've got you covered with tips applicable to any college year or comfort level. As you go throughout this chapter you will gain a better understanding of not only why different communities are important, but how to find, build, and sustain them, so that they ultimately have a positive impact on your college experience.

You're already into your second semester of your freshman year, and while you have people you're friendly with, it still doesn't feel like you're connecting with them the way you did with your high school friends. You want to have that college experience that everyone talks about but going to campus events by yourself feels too embarrassing and intimidating.

You were beyond excited when your best friend was accepted into the study abroad program of her dreams, but now that she's been gone for a few months, it feels like there's no one around. The ten-hour time difference feels impossible, and there's no way you can afford a ticket to go visit her over spring break. How are you supposed to feel connected to campus with your other half so far away?

But looking back now, you see that there have been countless opportunities to meet others on campus—kickoff meetings, student union activities, peer mentoring— and more importantly, from the looks of some upcoming events, it's never too late to make these connections. There's a planning session just around the corner for a food festival that sounds appetizing, and you know you've got a recipe to share.

Introduction

Moving from high school to college, especially if it's far from home, can come as a bit of a shock to the system. Those who you relied on throughout high school may not be as readily available, and long-distance relationships of any kind can be difficult to maintain. Maybe you're used to having a tight-knit group of friends, family dinners, or teachers, church leaders, and family friends who all know you inside and out. But even after a semester at college, you realize it's a lot harder to build meaningful connections than you remember. You want people to lean on who are part of your college life, but how are you supposed to find, build, and foster the community that you need?

The first place to start is to consider what a community is and who makes up yours in college. Think about your community as a support system, an army of people there to tackle the big and small day-to-day issues that arise and help you grow into your own and push you to be the best version of yourself. Friends, counselors, peer-mentors, club members, and advisors are all examples of people who might take on this role. Forming and engaging with a community in college is beneficial for all parties involved. When your core group shares common values or passions, both of you have the opportunity to grow and work toward something greater than yourselves. From offering support to teaching you new skills, there are endless ways in which community relations can have a positive impact on your college experience.

The types of communities you seek and the needs you want met are not going to be exactly the same throughout your life; it might not even be the same during the span of your college years. After you understand what type of community you're seeking—such as spiritual, social, academic—commit to enjoying the trial and error process. This means going to activity and club fairs, talking with professors and classmates, and more. See what happens when you truly open yourself up to welcoming others into your life. You might end up with a new best friend or a lifelong mentor!

Types of Communities

The reality is, no matter what campus you are at, you can find people you click with and faculty that will support you as you grow. While letting people in is fundamental to building meaningful relationships, it's also important to respect your boundaries and those of others. One way to make sure that you approach community building in the right way is to separate your communities in terms of those who are there for career and academic purposes and those who you want to fill social and personal needs. Here are some different groups of people you might find on campus.

I was fortunate enough to find many friends who were like-minded, regarding personal identity, goals, humor, and passions. I also worked to develop strong, bilateral relationships with my professors, so that I could gain a broader understanding of the curriculum while not feeling as overwhelmed.

— *Zachary, Occidental College*

Personal and Social Communities

If you are in your first year of college or transferring to a different school, one of the biggest adjustments can be making new friends. Joining a new peer group can feel impossible when you attend a university with over 30,000 students. Alternatively, it can be intimidating at a really small school if you feel like all 1,200 students are going to know everything about you. Don't overthink it! Your peers in college have the ability to provide support, friendship, and community, and they're all looking for a connection, too. Plus, there's a lot you can learn from them!

> Getting to know the people that lived around me helped me as well. Everyone is nervous as a freshman so don't be afraid to approach your peers as they may have the same gripes and fears as you. This is an opportunity to make new friends and network with people from vastly different cultures and upbringings.

—Stephan, University of Massachusetts, Amherst

The beauty of college is that you will be able to find like-minded peers, but also meet people from all different backgrounds. Both can be extremely helpful for your growth and your well-being. As you navigate new social situations, classes, and experiences, you'll have opportunities to find peers with similar interests and values. For example, Rachel at the University of California, Davis, wanted to have a strong Jewish community on campus. She checked out the university's Hillel House and began attending weekly shabbat dinners. If you keep considering your needs, you'll be able to identify those who will best make up your close-knit circle.

Your friend groups might shift a bit in college; that's normal. But it's nice to know there are always others out there who will support you, attend events with you, and just hang out with you if you're bored on a Saturday.

Fast Friends

Write down three things you want in a friend group.

1. _____

2. _____

3. _____

Academic and Career Communities

While in college, you're surrounded by a bevy of intellectuals including faculty, students, and more who are there to support you in all your academic endeavors. Not only are they a great source of knowledge and partners in innovation and curiosity, but they've been in your shoes and can help you be successful. Get involved in your academic community! There's strength in numbers, and the more people there are bolstering each other, the stronger the community will be.

Classmates

Your fellow classmates should also be included in your academic support circle. Having a study buddy or someone to share notes with you when you're sick can help you stay on top of your coursework and keep you both accountable. Upperclassmen in your degree program can even take on the role of a peer mentor. Just know when to wear your "school hat" and "friend hat."

Forming a group to share resources with (study guides, books, other miscellaneous things) can be really helpful!

—Maya, University of California, Berkeley

Professors

Professors can also play an important role in your time throughout college. Beyond the classroom, they may be the person who writes you a letter of recommendation for graduate school or a full-time job. They can recommend summer internship programs or research opportunities that will boost your resume or become a mentor. One of the easiest ways to gain access to professors is making the most out of your available interactions with them; that means attending their office hours and speaking up in class. Yes, it can feel annoying carving more time out of your day to attend office hours and speaking up in class can make you want to run the other way, but the more you do it, the more comfortable you'll get, and the more likely it is that your instructor will remember you.

Don't be afraid to talk to professors and ask questions! Many students fear asking questions, but it is honestly the best way to learn.

—Bridgette, Agnes Scott College

Most professors and teaching assistants will have accessible in-person office hours, but also online as well. Office hours are a great time to let them know about your professional ambitions. A lot of professors are also completing research in their respective fields, or are working professionals, and can offer insight into how your studies function outside the classroom. Make the effort to get to know your professors and learn from them.

Go to office hours and become friends with your professors, because they want you to succeed and will help you if they know you.

—Elizabeth, California State University, Northridge

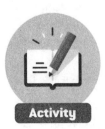

Office Hours Worksheet

Use this worksheet to prioritize and plan for meeting with instructors.

Class Name: _____

Instructor's Name: _____

Office Hour Location: _____

Time: _____

Write Down 3 Questions to Discuss (Homework, Internship Opportunities, Your Goals, Their Research, etc.)

_____

_____

_____

Write Down Their Responses

_____

_____

_____

Advisors

And if your classmates and instructors aren't enough, you can also include various advisors in your community for academic and professional support. Advisors can help you connect the dots between your education and your future career. Drop by their offices! They'll know how to make sure you're on the right path.

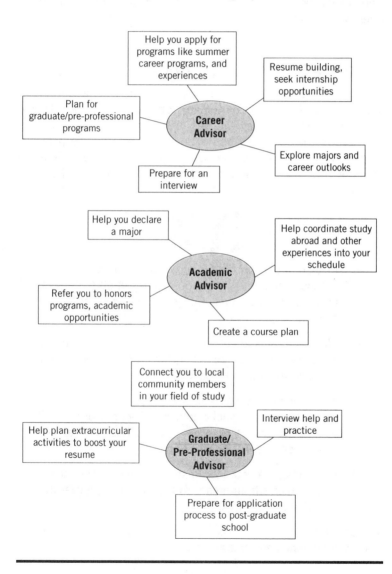

How Communities Can Help

Communities offer a variety of things; it's up to you to find the ones that most appeal to your gut and meet your needs. Perhaps you're looking for a group that makes you feel like you belong, or maybe you want to be around those that provide a sense of safety or stability. Maybe you want a group that you can stand out in, or one where you can fit right in when you're going through hard times.

Create a Sense of Belonging

Feeling like you belong helps to make you more confident in everything else that you do, not to mention fulfilled. You're more likely to take part in activities, navigate the nuances of campus, and make your forever friends. You'll be better equipped to handle potential hardships that may arise, like homesickness, which affects many first-year students. Here are some tips for how to make school feel like home, so you don't miss where you've come from (as much).

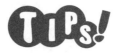

- Instead of only putting up pictures of your family and friends back home, try to add pictures of other things that bring you joy, especially things that you've discovered on campus.

- When you think about friends back home, try to put into words what you admire about them. Look for people on campus who match those key traits.

- Write one phrase that makes you feel bold, courageous, or just at peace. A sticky note with *I got this* or *you will accomplish great things* can be a reminder of what's to come even in a tough transition.

- If possible, ask your roommates to bring or cook their favorite meals from home. You can all connect over the food and the memories.

Remember that you're not alone. Everyone who is at college is starting something new right alongside you.

Provide a Feeling of Safety

Your health, safety, and well-being should be nonnegotiable to any community you're a part of. If they're not, and you cannot change those circumstances, you need to take steps to distance yourself from that group and find a better one. In some cases, issues can be resolved through conversations—for instance, if a person is making you uncomfortable at a party for the first time, ask them to stop. If they continue that unwelcome behavior, you may need to get others involved in removing yourself from any situations that involve them. Here are some ways to handle red flags:

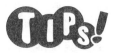

■ By all means, try new things in college, but do so because *you* want to do them. If you have any doubts, take a step back and consider your choices alone, without anyone whispering in your ear.

■ If you've blacked out or aren't sure what you did the night before, be very cautious about repeating the activities that put you there. If you've asked friends to watch out for you and they did not, carefully consider whether you can trust them with such a responsibility again.

■ You may find that some friends behave differently under certain circumstances. You can't necessarily change their behavior, but you can make a choice to not be around them when they make you uncomfortable. If you're concerned about their safety, make the time to talk with them in a neutral setting.

Value Individuality

In a school with thousands of students, it's easy to feel like your instructors don't know or really care about you, and you're just another body in a sea of undergrads. Don't let complacency fool you! There are plenty of faculty members, who, if you take the initiative, can have a lasting impact on you. They can serve as mentors in your studies, inspire you academically, and become allies, resources, and offer support when you need it. Not sure how to build up a relationship with your instructors? Here's some easy places to start.

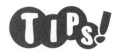

- Introduce yourself during their first week of office hours and continue going at least once a month to ask questions, discuss relevant current events, your ambitions, etc.

- Participate meaningfully at least once in every class.

- Attend their special lecture, reading, seminar, or whatever event they are putting on and speak to them after.

- When you need help, be honest and ask.

Go the Extra Mile

It can be hard to judge the strength of your community before it's been put to the test—there are plenty of people who will be there for you only when it's convenient, or when there's something in it for them. Keep this at the back of your mind when you're choosing the support that you keep around you. For instance, if you have the choice between two potential thesis advisors, think not only about which one can push you through a roadblock in your research, but which one will be there to help you step back and prioritize in the middle of a school-related panic attack. Are the friends who you associate with there because you share the same classes or study-abroad experiences, or would they also come over to lend an ear after a terrible break-up?

Keep in mind that in order for your relationship with these communities to remain healthy, you need to respect boundaries and engage with reciprocity. Boundaries can look like your roommate turning down an invite to hang out in favor of spending time alone to recharge, or your professor only wanting to meet during designated hours in their office. By valuing and knowing individual needs, you and the people you interact with can have much healthier and sustainable relationships. Additionally, be careful not to treat others solely as resources. While you want to be supported, so do others. If you only take and never give, your actions could be draining or harmful to others. Remember, everyone is looking to feel part of a community, so make sure that your behavior, in both the good and bad times, is reflective of the type of people you want to surround yourself with.

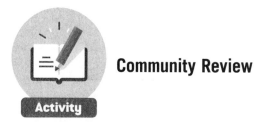

Community Review

Pick any local or campus event to attend and leave a review for it here. You can love it, or you can hate it, but get out there and evaluate how you felt about it afterward to help you find your place. Fill in the event and host details and color in the hearts to indicate how much you enjoyed yourself.

Event Name

♡ ♡ ♡ ♡ ♡

Event Host: _____ **Group Type:** _____

Services Provided (draw a ✔ or an ✗ next to each):

❏ Fun time	❏ Approachable people
❏ Good conversation	❏ Sense of belonging
❏ Acceptance	❏ Safe Space
❏ Learned something new	❏ Felt Included
❏ Added value to my academic and future career goals	❏ Would attend again

Highlights from the Event/Group:

1. _____

2. _____

3. _____

Write Your Review:

Where to Search for a Community

So where are you supposed to find these great people that change your life in college? Is it like every romcom that says you'll find love when you least expect it? Sure, you could just hit it off with the stranger who also sits in the hall between your Tuesday/Thursday class, but you can also actively seek out others who have shared interests, values, and goals. Keep reading for good places to start!

Clubs and Activities

Most colleges will have a club fair, typically at the beginning of each school year or semester, where all the clubs are out at tables with information about their club. You can walk around, grab some flyers, meet a few people, and get a date to attend the next club meeting to see if it is a good fit. If walking up to people at a giant fair immediately gives you anxiety, there are plenty of resources online for you to see what clubs and organizations are active, what the mission statements are, and how to contact them. You can typically find social media pages as well that give you more insight to what events are planned, the message and purpose of the club, and more. There are hundreds of clubs and organizations on college campuses that range in topics; you're bound to find something worth trying. Take a look at some of the most popular choices.

Academic

Academic clubs can help boost your resume, network with peers in your major, and help you with your coursework. Check for honors societies. Honors societies can be a way for you to earn scholarship money, receive recognition and awards, attend lectures in your academic area of interest, and even get published as a student. Especially if you're planning on applying to graduate/professional school, academic clubs can showcase interest in a specific discipline, which is added bonus points on your application!

Religious and Spiritual

Religious and spiritual organizations can offer a way for you to connect with others, whether that be to strengthen your own faith and interests or to explore other backgrounds. Check out spaces on campus like Hillel, churches, prayer and meditation rooms, gardens, and make note of when meetings are held.

Sports and Recreation

Sports and recreation clubs include intramural sports where you can participate with other students, stay active, have some healthy competition without being a recruited athlete. Options range from ultimate frisbee, crew, clogging, live action role play with Dungeons & Dragons, and more.

Issue- and Mission-Driven Clubs

There are many different clubs and organizations that put important issues or missions not only at the forefront of their activities,
but work on making it a priority on campus. Such activities include
political clubs, social justice clubs, multicultural student unions,
and LGBTQ+ clubs.

Special Interest Clubs

If you need a hobby or just like quirky activities, odds are there's a
club for that, too. Maybe you love trivia or cooking, or maybe you
just want to hang out with dogs. You can probably find something
that matches your special interest!

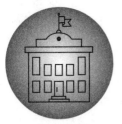

COLLEGE SPOTLIGHT
Northwestern University has a happiness
club with a mission to make others smile
while providing random acts of kindness
throughout campus. Their social media
page is filled with positive messages and
events including movie nights with s'mores,
Halloween pet costume contests, chicken
nugget nights, hugs and hot chocolate, and even a pie your professor
event.

Club Fair Scavenger Hunt

Activity

Head over to your school's club fair or activity website and write down the winners for each category!

Most fun:_____

Nicest people: _____

Least expected: _____

Most likely to get you out of your comfort zone: _____

Most adventurous: _____

Funniest idea: _____

One I'd be most likely to attend: _____

Most likely to boost my resume: _____

Most likely to bring a friend:_____

Most physically active: _____

Residential Housing and Campus Events

Residential housing events are a great place to meet your neighbors (and your neighbor's friends if they bring them!). Part of an RA's duties is to plan events and foster a sense of a community. It's a great way to explore campus, enjoy an activity, meet people who live near you, and often pick up some free food! There's nothing to lose at these casual and fun events. At the beginning of new terms, RAs often organize trips and floor contests to get students involved. If there's a trip taking your floor to the closest beach, hike, or outing to explore the city, take advantage! One trip might get you out of your comfort zone, or help you connect with someone new. Exchange phone numbers and room numbers so that you can grab dinner together or meet up another day.

Campus events bring together students of all different years and majors, so you're bound to meet new people while attending. Whether you're participating in a campus tradition, attending a Welcome Week concert, or cheering on your team in the student section, there will be someone you don't know who you have something in common with!

Department Events

Professors are a great way to get some academic guidance, but did you know you can connect with some who you haven't even taken a class from? Sounds obvious, but it's an easily forgotten trick you can use to not only learn a lot, but to inspire you academically! Look up professors who teach subjects or have backgrounds that you're interested in and ask to drop by their office hours to talk about their research or the field. Alternatively, a lot of colleges will host lunch or coffee meetups with professors and academic advisors, so you can attend one of these pre-organized events. Given that instructors also do their own research or writing, keep your eye out for speaker series and seminars that give you access to professors and experts beyond just attending class. Departments always have something going on, so don't let these opportunities slip by!

REFLECTION

How do you feel at the thought of becoming a part of various new communities? What steps can you take to boost your confidence as you try to integrate yourself into your college community?

_____

_____

_____

What do you need most from your communities? How do you make sure you're supporting others in your community?

_____

_____

_____

How comfortable are you researching and knowing where you can find groups to be a part of? List three steps you can take to meet people at your college.

_____

_____

_____

CHAPTER 9

Campus

This chapter will help you discover your campus in a way that works for you, regardless of where you are or what situation you're put in. It's all about your surroundings and how to use them for your benefit and your safety. First, we'll help you play tourist and research your new home in ways you may never have thought of, and give you tools to help you address a living environment you don't love. You'll use your surroundings to help break up monotony, get out of your comfort zone, and even find ways to boost your confidence along the way. This chapter will also address safety. Giving you the tools to prepare, plan, and manage a scenario that isn't in your favor, whether that's something big like a campus-wide emergency, or personal, like a situation needing exiting.

You're at a small university situated near a quaint town that has a few shops, a lot of scenery, and everyone knows your name. You hop on your bike and drop off a package at the one post office in town that happens to sit on your campus (because campus is practically the town). While you usually enjoy this routine and love your school, if you have to see yet another movie at the student union or ride along the same trail for the millionth time, you might go insane. Where can you get a little hustle and bustle and variety that you've been craving?

Living on a floor with other students in the honors program was going to be a great way to help you stay focused and keep your grades up while meeting people in your program. But after a few weeks, you're still not quite clicking with your roommate and no one ever takes you up on your invitation to go play some ultimate frisbee and snack on pizza. Coming back to your dorm feels stressful and lonely, rather than welcoming and relaxing. How are you supposed to deal with this for the rest of the year?

Partying has never really been your thing. You love to be social, and the thought of a big university seemed so appealing, but now that you're here, you're finding it hard to fit in without drinking. You know eventually you'll find your friends, but right now, it feels impossible without pretending to be something you're not. You miss home, you miss your friends who thought going to the local theater was fun, but most of all, you miss feeling under-stood. You're the life of the party, normally, just not this kind of party. So you pass up another invitation and choose a new show to binge on your laptop, feeling a bit deflated.

Introduction

If someone dropped a pin on your college campus on a map app, what would they see? Would it be a dot in a field of green, with just a single main road winding its way to the entrance, or would it be a dot lost in the middle of a city's classic gridlock pattern? Flip to street view, and you might see groups of students gathering in the quad outside their stone dorms that look like they were built in the 1950s or blurry pictures of buses, subway signs, and cars outside what might be a dorm, but also might just be office spaces.

Location plays a big role in your college experience. It's the type of area you live in, the place you wake up in every day, the environment you surround yourself in for a number of years. The beauty of college is that all campuses are unique in their own light. Each university has a different feel, and no two cities or towns are identical. Surely on some level, location, size, and campus feel played a role in your college selection process, but now that you're here, you might not know how to turn this town into your new home, especially if you have no idea how to get around or the adjustment has just not been what you expected. And while you may have known you wanted a specific environment for certain reasons, like a big city to land great internships, maybe you're really someone who prefers and yearns for peace, quiet, and grass. There's got to be a way to get the best of both worlds.

Every once in a while, it's good to pause and take a moment and widen your lens. Your college town may feel like a bubble or the city you find yourself in may be massive and all-consuming. Opening your perspective and allowing yourself to appreciate the good in your zip code (yes, there's something wonderful about every single area!) and to identify ways to escape when you need it will make you feel less constrained or homesick.

We often think of a place in terms of what you see on a map and how many people take up that space, but a place is also a feeling. Everyone wants to be at home in the world, so if you're thriving in your classes, but feel invisible as you walk through campus or wound up when you return to your dingey dorm with the roommate you can't stand, settling in can be challenging. Especially if your environment makes you feel unsafe, such external factors take an extensive toll on your mental health. But even though you can't change how big your school is or an unexpected emergency or uncomfortable situation that pops up, there are elements within your control that can help you turn these major stressors into something more amenable and safe for you.

Location

Whether you're 20 minutes from home or 2,000 miles away, you're in a whole new world and it's time to make it your own. When you researched colleges you might have had someone ask you what your ideal college climate would be. Rural, urban, or somewhere in between, and at that point, perhaps you just looked at your counselor or at the page in your guidebook and shared your preferences without hesitation. And even if you did hesitate, you made your choice, and now you're here. Sitting in between buildings, or nestled in a valley, you are here. So how do you use your living environment to your advantage? We'll help you master the art of living, regardless of where you are.

Always explore the area around your school. Whether that's paths in the forest next door (or in my case, a big, beautiful ravine), or city streets surrounding you, knowing what's outside the campus boundaries can help a lot with feelings of isolation.

—Annabel, Lewis and Clark College

Rural

You find peace in the smallness, the spaces that are quiet, serene, and make up the tight-knit community that becomes familiar. But what can you do when this environment is bringing you down? Here are some ways to shake things up, depending on how you're feeling:

I'm Isolated

- **Get Involved with the Local Schools**—Did you know that only 59% of graduates from rural high schools go to college in the fall? Whether this comes from a barrier to entry or feeling that college isn't even an option, you can find a way to work with current students and help build a relationship between the local high school(s) and your college. Not only will this be beneficial to your community, but you'll feel good about how you're spending your time, get out of your bubble, and feel grateful for the education you're receiving.

- **Talk with Locals**—Does your school get its food from a local farmer? Do you see the same server at the best food joint in town? Take some time to talk with these folks and get to know them as individuals. Everyone has a unique story that you can learn from. Who knows? Maybe you'll end up with a new job, a new friend, or at least an encouraging person behind you.

- **Make Time for that Trip**—We know that getting around can be challenging in rural areas if you have limited access to transportation. However, if you make the effort to plan out that adventure you've always wanted, you can have something special to look forward to, rather than feeling resentful that you can't go anywhere. Get friends involved, look into campus resources, and give yourself plenty of time to plan.

I'm Bored

- **Don't Knock It Till You Try It**—Alright, you're so over campus events: they all sound beyond corny to you. However, that "I'm too cool for this" mindset might be keeping you from having a good time with your fellow undergrads! Fear of looking goofy or getting out of your comfort zone isn't a reason to turn down a chance to kick back. Set a timer and an exit strategy: if you aren't having fun after giving it an earnest effort, leave!

Campus

- **Organize Your Own Fun**—If there's something you want to do, take it upon yourself to make it happen! If you're dying for a game night or want to plan an evening where you try something from every restaurant from your tiny downtown area, all you have to do is set it up. Maybe the student union can help you make an event posting for other interested students, or you can use social media or study groups to reach out to your circle. Make your fun a reality!

- **Get Really Into a Hobby**—Whether you want to learn Spanish or become an excellent frisbee player, diving into a passion is a great way to spend your time, better yourself, and boost your mood. Throwing yourself into something you love will help you feel more fulfilled and confident in yourself.

I Have No Opportunities

- **Make Your Own**—Do you want to work on a school paper but there's none to be found at your college? Maybe you were hoping to intern at the student health center but that doesn't seem like a thing? Plan ahead and see if you can create the opportunity you want that others can take advantage of in the future. It's definitely more work, but it's favorable to build relationships between universities and the local community. Get in touch with your department head, student center, or advisor to see if they have a point of contact or if anyone has tried to do something like this. They're here to help and will most likely be excited that you're taking the initiative to create opportunities.

- **Network**—Your professors had lives before they became your professor, and they also have friends and colleagues with different experiences. Use your close-knit relationship with your instructors to build your own network. Let them know what you're interested in and what you're searching for, and see if they can connect you with anyone in the field.

- **Go Virtual**—These days, there are tons of things that you can do online. Whether that's making money as a tutor or volunteering for a crisis hotline, you can find resume-boosting things that can be done from anywhere, even your small campus.

Urban

You've dreamt of city lights for many years now, but what if you're feeling disenchanted with the city you're calling home now? Here's how to help you fall back in love with the city.

I Can't Think

The hustle and bustle was fun during orientation, but now it's car horns and alarms and fire trucks and people yelling all the time. If you're looking for some peace and quiet, there are some ways to get it.

- Invest in a pair of noise-canceling headphones to help you work, or find a creative ways to muffle street noise by adding rugs and draft guards.

- Rework your space at home, whether that's adding blackout curtains or facing your desk away from the street.

- If you need some respite, find the park that's frequented by locals rather than tourists or take a train to somewhere quieter.

- Notice times throughout the day when areas are busier. If business districts are closed on the weekend to workers, you might be able to snag a table at the café with limited distraction, or if you find getting up an hour early before commuters begin to hit the pavement is a quieter time, set your alarm!

I Can't Catch a Break

Are you feeling the pressure? You might feel like you're not only competing with your classmates but with everyone else who wants to "make it" in this big old city you're in. Instead of thinking how you can outperform others, be confident in how far you've come and choose when to grind and when to enjoy the stage you're in.

- Don't let the fast pace of an urban environment get to you! Life is not a rat race, take a moment to acknowledge what you've already accomplished.

Campus

- Take time to practice mindfulness to help keep you stay kind to yourself and honor the work you're doing.

- Remind yourself of the mecca you live in by acknowledging the opportunities in front of you. What excited you about the city in the first place?

- List the things you can do here in the city that you can't elsewhere.

I Can't Afford Anything

Suddenly you can't eat lunch out for less than $20, and you never thought laundry would be an expense to worry about. City living can be painful on the wallet, but luckily there are things you can do that won't break the bank.

- **Set a Budget**—instead of trying to do everything every day, plan to do one thing every week or month depending on your resources. You can treat this as a reward and make it something to look forward to as opposed to thinking of it as something you can't enjoy.

- **Look for Discounts**—Always look for student discounts, and stay in touch with your school, which might have its own arrangements with certain establishments for free events or group rates.

- **Find Free Things**—While it's true that individual activities may be more expensive in a city environment, there are also likely to be way more activities offered. And when you stop looking at the cost of one specific thing, you may find free alternatives and trials if you can, say, wait until Tuesday night to go to a museum, or Saturday morning to see a film.

Suburban

Suburban campuses, or campuses that are somewhere in between urban and rural, afford the luxury of being a part of a traditional college feel, meaning your campus boundaries are clear and you're not lost in the shuffle. The student bodies can vary in size, but you feel fairly confident in navigating campus as a whole. These college campuses can present a unique set of frustrations that overlap with both rural and urban campuses.

You can expect a suburban area to be primarily residential, with local parks filled by neighborhood toddlers and parents. Dining options may lean more toward chain restaurants, and local entertainment is not only less likely to be within walking distance but might not be near any public transportation. Don't worry, you can still get creative.

I Still Feel Stuck

- If it seems like there's just one bus that runs sporadically and rarely in your favor, make sure you're tapped into the bus schedule and show up early so you don't miss the rare ticket out. To avoid getting trapped, reach out to your friend groups to find those with cars, and offer to share expenses for excursions.

- The local scenery might be tailored more towards family lifestyle, but that doesn't mean you can't take advantage of the spaces. See if you can access and rent community parks and recreation centers; these can be good places to change things up with club meetings or intermural practices.

- Every neighborhood tends to have its own benefits and discounts: keep an eye out for opportunities unique to your area, like a bowling alley with a young adult league. Grab your friends and don't be afraid to shake it up a bit!

I Feel Misplaced

- When students make up a small part of a neighborhood, it can seem difficult to find an opportunity. But on the flip side, there are likely fewer applicants with your credentials for those postings in your area—and being a local can help.

- Just because something isn't listed, doesn't mean it's not there. Step up your networking game and ask local community organizations if they have any positions open, or a need for help. Any professors who live in the area can likely offer some specific guidance.

- If your campus feels like a commuter campus, get to know people living in on-campus housing and begin attending university events. The events might feel silly at first, but you're all in this together, so no shame in attending a late-night pizza event, especially if you're bored!

Regardless of where you are, it's your job to seek the things that bring you joy and think out of the box when you feel bored or disconnected. You have the power to find the peace in the business and find the busy in the quiet and to play tourist and find the local gems that are outside of the guidebook.

Where Are You?

Answer the following questions:

What type of campus environment are you in? (city, close to city, rural/remote, etc.)

_____

What is one space off campus that you find peace, or a moment to unwind?

_____

What's one place you'd like to explore outside of campus?

_____

What's one place you've been to that brings you joy, productivity, and/or support?

_____

Playing Tourist

You can't know what you've got until you've actually seen it. Research on the neighborhood can help, to a point, but only if others have written about it and, more importantly, if you share the same mindset as the writer. Better still to become an expert yourself by trying out the so-called "best croissants in town." If you feel stuck in a rut, explore a bit, whether that's walking through a nearby park, taking a bus to a new nook of town, or taking a train an hour down the coast to see something new.

Do Your Research

Get on Google maps, type in your university, and zoom out. Get your bearings. If it's your first year, just looking at a map will help you get a sense of what you have access to. Look for any greenery or bodies of water close by where you might be able to hang out or do some work. Running and walking trails are often synced in the maps as well, so you can look for some mileage whether you need to break a sweat or the monotony of a rough day.

When you find something you like, take note of the various ways to get there, especially if you're not used to public transportation routes in your area. If you're hesitant about exploring new places, use the street view to get familiar with what buildings look like and write out directions so do you don't have to be glued to your phone the whole time and can be more aware of your surroundings.

Look up online guides and blogs detailing everything from the best landmarks and parks to the best noodles in town. Get lost in a sea of tabs with recommendations from people who've already explored the area and save the sites you prefer. Look at online reviews, chat with your friends who are local to the area, and use social media to your advantage. Follow local restaurants and the city's/town's social media pages to stay up-to-date on events and snag some discounts.

Campus

Get Out There

Done your research? It's time to fly. Okay, maybe not fly, but at least get out there. First, it's okay to acknowledge that we all have our different routines and avenues for exploring. So maybe you're a creature of habit, that's fine! But you still have the ability to find the places that bring you some comfort. Second, be open and try a few places. Perhaps you pick a different block or area every month to explore. Or participate in a seasonal event, like a strawberry festival or a 5K in the city center. Don't be embarrassed to do corny "overrated" things. You're looking for new experiences to help you bond with your town. Grab a friend if you want someone to keep you more likely to commit to the event. Either way, participating in a community event can help fight feelings of isolation and open doors to new possibilities.

Residential advisors will often organize local outings either by bus or walking, especially at the start of a term. You might find yourself on a black sand beach at the basin of a forest you had no idea existed, or on a nature walk where you learn about the state flower and take in the new scenery. All you're committing to is a few hours of your time, if you hate it, well you're still learning about yourself and what you don't need, so get out there and try something new. You never know what you'll find.

Be Friendly

If you're in a completely different state, or just new to the area, get to know students who can show you the ropes whether that's a student who's already from the state, or an older student who's been there for a few more years. Eventually, you'll find your groove and what works for you, but the benefit of being open to new experiences and advice from others is learning about hidden gems not easily found online. If you frequent the same sandwich shop, ask for recommendations while you wait. Locals can give you inside information like the best time to take the subway, or the discounted theater showing classic movies for only five dollars on Tuesdays.

Or just grab a group of friends and head out on an adventure. Maybe you meet up with some friends from other universities within the same city. If they're alumni from your high school or old friends, it can be nice to catch up with familiar faces. You meet at the farmer's market, central to all of your campuses, you walk through grabbing goodies, swap stories of painful professors, reminisce about the past, and share plans for Thanksgiving break.

I spend a lot of time in and around Tempe, Phoenix, and Scottsdale. A lot of my friends are from the area so they show me around. It's really healthy for my mind to get a break from being in the same place.

—*Dan, Arizona State University*

Follow Your Comfort Level

Depending on what year you are, how much you know the area, and where you are, nothing matters as much as you going at your own speed. If you're someone that likes to take your time getting comfortable with your surroundings at a pace that doesn't feel rushed, that's fine!

Look, we get it, exploring a new environment can be a bit over-whelming. Especially if you're more of an introvert, or just exhausted. Keep in mind, there will be days where you just don't feel like going out. That's perfectly okay. But you can come up with creative ways to take yourself out of your comfort zone. After all, college is about growth and part of that is acclimating to and exploring new and different situations.

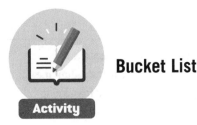

Bucket List

Activity

There's nothing like a bucket list to keep you motivated to get out of your comfort zone and try something new! Research what's around you and fill in one bucket list item for each category. Have fun with it!

Off-campus adventure	
An event	
Local restaurant you've always wanted to try	
Campus tradition	
One outdoorsy excursion	

Housing

For many first-year students, college is the first time they're living away from home. It can be tricky enough to adjust to dorm life or eventually figure out what the difference is between on-campus and off-campus apartments. But throw in dealing with roommates or accommodations that don't quite meet your expectations, and that space that's supposed to be your stress-free haven for sleeping, studying, and socializing can quickly become a source of constant frustration.

Finding the Right Housing

Maybe when you were selecting your first-year housing, you felt rushed or just went in blind. Perhaps you had limited options as a freshman, and now you can choose from all sorts of accommodations and don't know where to begin. No matter your circumstances, there are many tools to help you figure out what the right housing situation is for you.

Research Your Campus Options

Depending on where you attend, there are several types of accommodations you can end up in. Dorms, suites, singles, student apartments, or even Greek housing options are all unique. Some housing choices mean you'll be required to have a meal plan or share a room with someone, while others come fully equipped with a kitchen. The best way to figure out which one is right for you is to do your research on what's out there, what you qualify for, and keep track of your priorities.

Get online and dive into the housing websites for each of the campus options. They usually list basic info like set up, cost, and amenities. This is a great way to compare and narrow down your choices. However, we highly suggest taking a tour of any place before you move in. Most colleges offer tours of their housing, or you can ask around and try to find someone who lives in the place you're interested in.

Campus

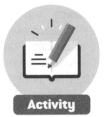

Housing Priorities

Activity

In the center, write down your top priorities, or, if you have them, non-negotiables. Then, draw an arrow to the best type of housing that matches your preferences. Include things like location, cost of rent, square footage, noise level, preferred number of roommates, etc. in your priorities.

1. Apartment

3. Dorm

_____

_____

_____

_____

_____

2. Community

4. Greek House

Living Learning Communities

In regard to your living situation, if you're about to head off to college, check out the available living learning communities in the dorms. Read more about a specific community, ask an admission counselor, or a university representative for more information. Talk to current students within the living learning community for their perspective on pros and cons. If the living learning community is honors-based and you're interested, check out the requirements for qualifying, review application timelines, and submit an application. You might need letters of recommendation or a minimum GPA. Even if you're in your sophomore year in college, there can be an opportunity to join an honors college, that might provide some more opportunities academically and socially, so check it out.

Roommate Matching

Does finding someone to live with stress you out? Does living with a total rando elevate your blood pressure? You're not alone! Cohabitating, especially in close quarters, is a major adjustment for everyone. However, you do have options. If you can live with pretty much anyone, you can certainly choose to go with a random roommate assignment if offered for your housing choice. Alternatively, you can go through your school's matching page or a third-party site to find someone who is a good fit for your lifestyle, housing preferences, and personality. Sometimes "matching services" take a more informal tone with students asking friends if they have friends who are also searching. Get creative! People are always coming and going on college campuses, so odds of you finding someone to live with are high.

Exploring Off-Campus

Off-campus housing comes with its own stressors separate from campus housing. Luckily, you can learn a lot from this experience and apply it to looking for housing even after college. Here are some basic questions to ask when doing a tour of an off-campus apartment:

- What is the lease term?
- What is included in the rent?
- How much are utilities?
- Are there any additional fees (broker fees, pet fees, etc.)
- What is the laundry situation?
- Is parking available?
- How is maintenance handled?

Make sure that before you sign a lease, that you read it through thoroughly and ask questions if you have them! Additionally, many schools have services to help students read through their lease and understand how the housing market works in your area.

Living with Roommates

Even if you do your due diligence finding a roommate, you're probably going to have a conflict at some point. That's OK! You have options in when it comes to dealing with living differences. Try these out the next time something comes up and see how it goes for you.

Voice Your Concern

As much as you wish it were true, your roommate probably cannot read your mind. If they never shut off their alarm clock or keep forgetting to lock the door when they leave, and it drives you bonkers, let them know nicely. Whenever possible, try to have this conversation in person. Use a respectful tone, keep it brief and light, and be clear with the problem. If you can, try to pose a solution! For example, you might say, "Thanks for taking a minute to chat with me. I just wanted to talk about keeping our room clean. Instead of letting the trash overflow, would you be open to taking turns each week to empty it?"

Learn How to Compromise

Sometimes, conflicts require concessions on both sides. Maybe your roommate is dating a new guy, and he's over every single weekend Friday through Sunday. The space is small as it is, and now you're having to worry about walking in on them or not being able to relax in your space during your only free days. When working to compromise with someone, make the effort to know your boundaries, while also putting yourself in their shoes. For example, you might let your roommate know you're excited for their budding relationship and desire to spend time with their new partner but suggest that instead of him coming to your dorm every weekend, maybe they alternate weekends so you can still enjoy your space.

RA Mediation

If you have tried voicing your concerns and handling roommate conflict on your own, sometimes you need to bring in back up. This is especially true if you're dealing with illegal activities like underage drinking or drug use. Your RA is there to help! Bringing in a third party to help mediate a tougher or more serious situation can take some of the stress off you.

Moving

Sometimes the best way to solve roommate issues is to move. If you've done what you can and it's still like trying to fit a square peg into a round hole, it's time to look into alternative options. Talk with campus housing about what's involved with making a switch and how to get that ball rolling. Note, if you're trying to leave an off-campus situation, it is generally much more challenging (and expensive!) to break a lease, so be sure to look through that contract and what type of freedom you have in regards to moving or subletting.

Transportation

If you're uncomfortable getting around or feel unsafe, it's definitely going to prevent you from going out to do things you enjoy or being social with friends. There's a seemingly endless number of services provided, such as buses, trains, subways, rideshares, and more. Here's what you need to know about getting from point A to point B.

How to Navigate

Knowing how to get around can feel liberating. When you're not intimidated by a map or know the best method for getting around, you'll be a lot more willing to do the things you want to do. To start, get to know the services you're close to and would use consistently, like the subway. Download an app so that you can keep up with timetables, service interruptions, and plan out routes. As you keep riding the same routes, it'll start to become second nature.

For a one-off trip or occasional outing, it's good to do some research beforehand. If you have a specific destination in mind, check their website to see if they offer a recommended route or provide directions. Your RA or someone at the student union might also be able to provide you with information about car rental discounts for students, rideshare services, shuttle buses to the airport, and more! You'll never know if you don't ask, so go ahead and find out what your school has in place to help you get around.

Staying Safe

When getting around, you want to stay alert to your surroundings and make sure you're following best practices to keep yourself safe.

Here are our tips to help you feel and stay safe:

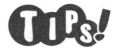

- Use a stop that is well-lit and in a relatively active area.
- Don't stand too close to the road or platform edge when waiting.
- Travel with someone when possible.
- Plan ahead and know your route.
- Don't sleep in the bus, subway, taxi, etc.
- Always confirm your driver's car and name before entering a Lyft, Uber, etc.
- Have your fare handy.
- Hold onto your belongings at all times.
- Don't engage in unnecessary conversation with strangers or give out personal info.
- If someone makes you feel uncomfortable, get out of the car or move seats.
- Never get in a car with someone who you think is intoxicated.

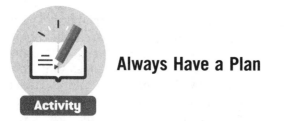

Always Have a Plan

If you've been putting off an activity because you're anxious about getting there and back, plan the whole thing out.

Destination: _____

Possible Routes (Research!):

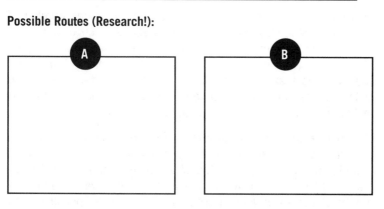

Public Transportation Hours of Operation: _____

Friends Going to Event: _____

Cab Contact Information and Cost: _____

Finalized Plan: _____

_____

Size

The physical size of your campus can be a blessing working in your favor, but it can also turn into a nightmare if you're feeling stuck, or just a bit lost. A big school at first feels amazing, with plenty of things to do and explore, but if you're overwhelmed with social situations and can't find your own kind of fun, it loses its appeal. Finding your way in a new campus is an art, not a science. Follow these tips to help you get acclimated no matter the size of your school.

Big School

There are many advantages to a big college, from the number of available experiences to the often roaring sense of school spirit. But that size can also make it take longer for everything to click into place. For starters, if you're at a big school, just learning how to find your way and make friends takes a minute. It's often a solid year or two before you find your people and your type of fun, and start feeling like you're a part of something.

Use your campus to your advantage. If you don't fit in one hundred percent because Greek life isn't your thing or you're not that big of a drinker and it seems that's the only draw for fun, it can definitely make you feel stressed. While hiding under your covers and binging the latest season of your favorite TV show sounds appealing (and yes, that is still something you can do), don't give up on finding your people and your way in a big school.

For starters, you're not the only one feeling this way. Get involved with activities and find like-minded people who have the same ideas about fun. If you do end up at a party and just don't feel like drinking, diffuse an awkward conversation by saying something simple and clear like, "I don't feel like drinking tonight" and then change the conversation. People are likely to follow your lead or tone in a conversation so if you keep it light and move on, odds are they will too. This is even easier if you're with a buddy who feels similarly to you, as two people can more easily drive a conversation away from boundaries they're uncomfortable with.

Medium School

You're at just the right school. Not too big and not too small. So everything's easy, right? Well, maybe not. Some of the same stressors might apply as well as some new ones. Perhaps a majority of the student body comes from the local community and you feel like everyone already knows each other. The student body feels one-note and the ones that have been there for some time don't hang around after class, let alone the weekends. You'd like to get into town, but the amenities, while vast, are sparsely spaced. Your classes aren't as consistent and while stereotypes are never your thing, it can be hard to pinpoint where you might fit in.

A medium school provides opportunity for you to put yourself out there with a little less intimidation. You're likely to find new friends, even if you attend an event and realize it's not your scene, and you have a smaller sense of community even if it doesn't feel like it right now. Getting picky about the things you value and your ideas of fun, will help you feel more confident in finding groups of friends who feel the same.

Small School

In a small school, the community can feel close-knit and supportive, and your campus can easily become your own, however, it can also feel a bit monotonous. For starters, maybe you want a more diverse student body and you feel like an island. "Everyone's got their cliques, no one really understands where I'm coming from." If you've been attending a small college for a while now and still feel like you haven't found your people, it can feel even more alone.

As cliche as it sounds, you have the ability to change how you view the world around you. Your perspective on anything can have a direct impact on how you feel. If you're feeling isolated and completely out of touch from your university experience, turn inward and really think about how you can adjust your outlook. What's in your control? If you're feeling like the only student from a specific background, this might mean vocalizing to your friends that you feel your perspective is disregarded. While it is not your responsibility to educate others about struggles or oppressions you've faced, you can protect yourself by making note of and reporting any types of acts or microaggressions that make you feel unwelcomed.

If you're looking specifically for other students with a shared background or experience, continue to seek out events, clubs, and opportunities that do so. You might even consider creating a space on your own and find that many others were looking as well. Making campus inclusive goes two ways. If you are someone who fits the mold of a typical student at your school, always check yourself to make sure your behavior is inviting to all and speak up when you see someone who is left out, disregarded, or otherwise mistreated. Making an inclusive atmosphere can be challenging, but it's essential to creating the best campus experience possible.

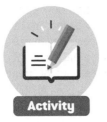

Activity

In Your Own Words

In your own words, define the following terms as they relate to how much you feel like a part of your campus.

Acceptance_____

_____

Belonging _____

_____

Exclusion _____

_____

Home _____

_____

How good am I at helping others feel they belong?

○ 1   ○ 2   ○ 3   ○ 4   ○ 5

This is	This is
hard for	easy for
me	me

How strong is my sense of belonging in my school today?

○ 1   ○ 2   ○ 3   ○ 4   ○ 5

This is	This is
hard for	easy for
me	me

Campus

My goal for acclimating to campus this week:

_____

_____

_____

Strategies to help me reach my goal:

_____

_____

_____

_____

Safety

You're on your own. Getting to know your surroundings and resources is imperative to remaining safe not to mention preparing ahead of time so your body knows what to do when your mind shuts down in an emergency. We'll walk you through potential scenarios and provide tips to get you through whatever comes your way.

Campus Safety

You've been studying late at the library, or visiting with friends, and you find yourself having to return home in the dark. Perhaps the campus feels empty and unsettling. Well, it's important to remember that your school has its own campus security, as well as safety features that you can access. Here are some ways to be proactive and feel comfortable at school regardless of the hour.

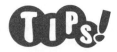

- If you're driving, make a point of parking in a higher-traffic area so that it's easier to get back to your car afterhours.

- If you can meet up with a friend, or leave with them, it can be a comfort to not be alone, especially as you're getting acclimated to a new area.

- If you can't be with a friend in person, consider asking one of them to keep you company on the phone. Mind you— this isn't the time for a deep conversation, as you need to be listening to what's going on around you, especially while crossing streets. But knowing that a friend knows where you are can be stress-relieving.

- Have what you need at hand before you set out. This not only means having objects like pepper spray, keys, or phone easily accessible, but also means knowing exactly where you're going so that you can pay attention to the environment as you walk.

- Use the blue-light emergency posts if you need to reach campus security directly; you can also check for download-able apps or phone numbers that can do the same.

■ See if your campus offers any door-to-door escort services that can pick you up and drive you directly to another on-campus area.

In short, be aware of your surroundings, be alert about what's happening on campus, and know where to go in the case of an emergency.

Party Safety

You're at a party, you're not loving the scene, you've lost your friends, your phone is about to die, and it hits you that you have no idea how to get back home. College can bring some uncomfortable scenarios in social settings. How do you get by? For starters, make a plan ahead of time. Go to parties or places with people you trust. Have a signal, stay connected, and make a plan for when you or someone else wants to leave. Especially if you're really uncomfortable, and want a quick exit, power in numbers can be beneficial. If you're drinking, protect your drink and know what cup is yours. You never want anyone pouring a drink for you that you're not aware of what's going in the cup. Know your limits and stick to them. You are never forced to stay in a situation you're uncomfortable in, so even if you have to lie, or say something as an excuse to leave, do whatever is necessary to safely leave.

Sexual Assault

According to the 2019 Association of American Universities survey polling over 150,000 students, on average, nonconsensual sexual conduct, sexual contact by physical force, or an inability to consent, was thirteen percent and more likely experienced by female students and undergraduate students overall. Sexual assaults on college campuses are often underreported as victims may feel ashamed, embarrassed, or not wanting to incriminate the perpetrator. Sexual violence can have long-term mental health effects. If you ever find yourself sexually assaulted you are not alone, and you have the ability to receive help by your university. Go to the campus health center for an exam and a trusted professional will help you with the steps to get help, including potentially filing a police report. There are also support groups and counseling services are also available for these situations. Get the support you need to feel safe. It is never your fault and never too small or too late to get help. You deserve to feel safe physically, mentally, and emotionally.

Emergency Plans

You've almost certainly had an emergency plan before. Maybe you didn't think it up yourself—it was the evacuation plan on the back of a bathroom door at an office building, or it was the fire drill at your high-school—but you knew what to do in the case of an emergency. Even if you scoffed at the directions, you probably got some measure of comfort from knowing how to react in the middle of a crisis.

Well there is actually something to that. Practice makes perfect. When you're in an emergency it can be hard to think clearly. Your heart's pounding, your brain's fuzzy, and you can be in a state of shock or panic. Whether it's an environmental disaster or a campus crisis, it's really important that you build muscle memory and a familiar response to an emergency, so your body just knows what to do. In a dorm, know where the exits are or in your apartment be aware of how to get out of the house. In both scenarios, have a back-up plan take a minute for you to check things like stairwells, windows, and think about how you would exit quickly, and safely. As you register and begin attending classes, pay attention to exits, pathways that get you back to your dorm, or to an open area in case of an emergency.

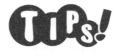

Keep a simple first-aid kit handy as well as an emergency kit which should include some of the following:

- Flashlight
- Pepper spray
- Some cash (particularly in smaller bills)
- Water
- Nonperishable food
- A blanket
- Extra batteries
- Gloves
- Masks
- Hand sanitizer
- Toilet paper

- Antibiotic ointment
- Bandages
- Matches
- Can opener
- Medicines for prescriptions

- Jacket/extra pair of clothes
- Whistle
- Hydrogen peroxide
- Alcohol wipes

In preparing for emergency situations, know also what to do in case of an active shooter. Active shooter situations can escalate quickly; it is vital to assess your surroundings and get yourself in a protected and locked position as best as you can. If you're in an open area, go to the nearest room, lock yourself inside, and get out of sight from any windows. Hide under desks, put your phone on silent so as to not make any noises, or show any lights. If you are in a bathroom where you cannot lock the main door to the entrance, lock yourself in a stall and kick your legs up against the door to your stall not showing any parts of your body. It can feel really scary, or just completely out of the realm of possibility to prepare yourself for an active shooter or any threat on campus, for that matter, but having a plan and knowing all surroundings and resources available is one of the best ways to keep yourself protected and ultimately alive.

Social Media Safety

Social media is amazing at connecting to friends and family wherever you are, getting to know a new crush through DMs, creating stories, exploring new feeds, and just scrolling your way through a boring class (we won't knock you for that!). However, it has its drawbacks, and safety can be at the top of that list. There are simple things you can do to protect yourself with your accounts. For starters, if you're tagging your location in real time wherever you are, and your account is public, anyone else can find you. Some photos may also automatically geotag your location, even if you haven't provided it. If you have any concerns about being followed, go into your privacy settings and turn off all location settings and consider making your accounts private. At the very least, set up different settings to where close friends or smaller groups of people you're comfortable with can see a majority of your posts, rather than it all open.

If you're on a site, or sending information to another person, never give out things like social security numbers or even student ID numbers, especially if it's not a school official or a verified source. Credit card companies or scammers can easily hack through your accounts with limited information, so be aware of what you're sharing and also change up your passwords every now and again. Stay away from unsecured wireless networks and if you're using multiple devices, log out of your accounts, and keep your passwords private and stored somewhere safe. You can use your phone for good and share your location with a trusted friend. If you're going on a date, heading to a party, or just were supposed to be home from class and have been missing, it's a good idea to have someone else aware of your whereabouts.

Social Media Consumption

Being safe with social media also includes your usage and monitoring the amount of time spent on apps. Think about how you feel after you're done scrolling. If you find yourself often comparing yourself to other accounts or you feel drained after browsing feeds instead of being energized and motivated, odds are what you're following isn't doing any favors to your mental health. Filters set you up for unrealistic expectations, so don't try to model expectations off the one person on your wall who always looks like they walked out of a catalog, doing incredibly well and just overall crushing it at life. No one is posting the fight they got into with their mom over the phone in the morning or the test they just failed, but it can be really hard to remember that when you're only ever seeing a carefully curated selection of best moments.

Set time limits on your consumption and if you find you need a little more support, use the settings on your phone that will block apps after a certain amount of time. Follow accounts that bring you joy and inspiration rather than negativity and mute/block peers that no longer serve you in a positive light.

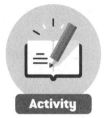

Activity

Emergency Contact List

Don't wait until the last minute to figure out who to contact. Put together a list of phone numbers and URLs that have the information you need in the event of any kind of help, whether that's for an emergency, or just for some help or reassurance on a class project.

Type of Contact	Name	Phone
Local Contact		
Out-of-State Contact		
Next of Kin or Family Member		
Work Contact		
Neighbor, Roommate, etc.		
Physician		
Other Emergency Contact		
Preferred Hospital		
Local Police Precinct		
Campus Police		
Fire Station		

REFLECTION

How comfortable are you exploring your college campus? What are three things that would motivate you to get out there?

_____

_____

_____

Consider a recurring issue (roommate drama, a busted radiator, etc.) you have in your current living situation. Write out a game plan for how to address it the next time it comes up.

_____

_____

_____

What is your preferred method of getting around campus? How do you feel about getting off campus when you need or want to? Explain.

_____

_____

_____

Identify one thing you're not particularly loving about your campus vibe right now. What's one active thing you can do to improve your setting or adjustment you can make?

_____

_____

_____

What is one area of safety you do not feel as equipped to handle? What are things you can do to feel safer? Whether that's making a plan, identifying a resource, or creating a buddy system, write it down and be specific.

_____

_____

_____

Campus

CHAPTER 10

Career

This chapter will introduce you to different career services potentially offered by your college and help you make the most of them. Regardless of where you are in college, this chapter will help assess your personal strengths, interests, values, and skills to help you as you navigate college majors and ultimately career choices. This chapter will discuss the ways career services can help and give you practical examples and tips for things like creating a strong resume and knowing how to network successfully. Use these tips and exercises to guide you towards the services that best fit your needs. Your career starts here!

What are your plans after graduation? asks your uncle, your neighbor, and pretty much every other adult you encounter while home over winter break. A few semesters ago, you felt that same sinking feeling in your stomach when asked about what you were going to study. Sometimes it might seem like as soon as you reach one milestone, you need to be charging down a well-laid path to the next big goal. You know you want a job and a career, but the mounting pressure and general uncertainty on what's out there and what you want to do is making you want to burst. *Oh I'm still weighing my options. Maybe grad school?* you answer, knowing fully well that you're not even sure if you want to dive right back into two to three more years of intensive studying.

It feels like every student around you has had some sort of an internship or at least some club experience, and you're quietly panicking that you barely feel confident in your major choice. You thought you knew what you wanted to do, but after some prerequisite classes, you feel completely misplaced. The idea of switching majors feels overwhelming, but so does sitting through classes disengaged as you watch your peers climb the ladder you feel trampled on. How will you ever catch up and get back on your career track?

Introduction

Choosing a university might have been stressful, but now that you're here, you've got bigger fish to fry. As you choose your classes and begin to carve out a more concrete plan of what to focus on, you'll eventually have to decide a major, maybe a minor or certificate, and ultimately a career. Maybe you're at the beginning of that road, where you have yet to declare a major, or maybe you've declared a major, but are now second guessing your choice. But even after you've chosen an area of study, you now have the job of standing out from your peers. Graduating with a degree is one thing but graduating with a degree and a handful of experiences such as internships, research, and job experience is another. You need guidance, and you need it sooner rather than later!

Luckily, that's why colleges have career services. While the future can be uncertain, many colleges have career services that can not only guide you in the right direction but get you excited and confident about what happens next. Yet somehow, these services can be one most students overlook. In fact, less than half of students even take advantage of campus career resources. But not you! You're going to join the ranks of those who took advantage of the available resources. While resources will vary between schools, this chapter will introduce you to some of the most common and well-used tools career centers offer, from resume support to networking events and more.

A career might seem like something you don't need or want to consider until the end of college. However, even though you might not know where to start, you're plain terrified, or the idea that you might "fail" at it is paralyzing, your college years are a great time to explore and prepare for possible job trajectories. Career services can help you explore your personal interests, strengths, and values, and work with you to find the right major, find extracurricular opportunities that expand your resume, and also prepare you for your first interview. Showing up is your first step to getting started, and when you show up for yourself, really great things can happen.

From Major to Career

There are dozens of majors to choose from, and some schools even let you design your own. If your major is supposed to lead to a certain job, how are you supposed to pick one if you don't know what you want to do for the rest of your life? Rest assured you're not alone in your anxiety. First, take a breath and remind yourself that there's value in each and every subject you can study. Your school wouldn't offer a degree in it otherwise! Next, refocus your energy to take a deep dive into learning about yourself. Why? Because taking the time to better understand your personality, values, and preferences can help you nail down the type of career path you ultimately want.

Assessing Yourself

Taking a personality assessment is a fun way to gain a better understanding of who you are and how you interact with the world around you. It is also helpful in finding your strengths and preferences for how you want to live your life. One popular assessment is the Myers-Briggs Type Indicator® (MBTI). You answer a number of questions that ask you about your preferences in different areas and at the end you receive a detailed report with a distinct personality type. From there, you are able to learn about your type and what scenarios you thrive best in. For example, you might learn you're an INFJ ("the Counselor") and have an affinity for helping others and choose to try out a major in social work. There are many different types of assessments beyond the Myers-Briggs tests, all with the goal of better understanding the traits that make you who you are! Check with your career office or an academic advisor to help access the assessments they have available, in the meantime, complete this quick activity to get you started!

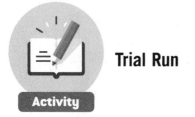

Trial Run

Activity

Write down all of your classes, extracurriculars, activities, and jobs from a semester of your choice below.

Next, add up the number of items you listed.   **Total Items:** _____

Now, score your items listed based on which one you liked the most. For example, if you have 5 classes and 2 activities, for a total of 7 items, your favorite will get 7 points, your second favorite 6, and so forth.

Using the same scoring system as above, consider each of the three career tracks below. Answer the following questions and assign points to each track to indicate your interest in that path. The track with the most points should be the trajectory that interests you the most.

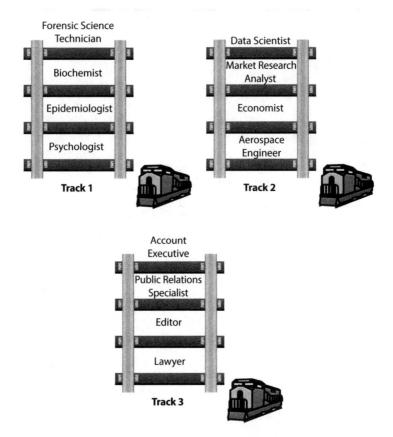

1. What stood out most about the class or extracurricular you assigned the highest score?

   _____

2. How does your highest ranked class or extracurricular from Part I relate to the track you chose on Part II?

   _____

3. Name one thing you can do to advance toward the career track you think you're interested in.

   _____

Valuing Yourself

Knowing what you value is another way to gain some clarity. Values are essentially fundamental beliefs and attitudes that influence your decisions and actions. Your values may change over time and that is okay, but as you consider major and career choices, it is helpful to check in with your values to see if the two align. For example, if you value creativity and autonomy, you might consider studying art history and business so you can open your own gallery. Alternatively, maybe community and purpose are important to you, and you work with the career center to find an internship that focuses on social justice.

By looking at your values in relation to both the short-term (your major or minor) and long-term (your career), you're setting yourself up for a more fulfilling path. Exploring your values can lead you to try out different courses, participate in unique research or study abroad opportunities, and explore internships or volunteer work that not only help you make progress toward your major, but help you find a field in which you can see yourself working.

Ask the Experts

While it's good to imagine how you might do in hypothetical career scenarios based on various assessments during college, you have access to upperclassmen, faculty, and alumni who can speak to you about their real life major to career experiences. Informational conversations can help you determine if the demands of a major or job trajectory is something that excites you. You might find others have had the same fears that you do and gain tips on how they overcame obstacles. In addition to on-on-one meetings, see if departments are hosting a seminar, job fair, or alumni networking night within your specific discipline. These are great ways to learn about possible career paths, make connections, and learn more about what fields you enjoy (or don't!).

Career

Save the Date

Prioritize learning about potential majors and career paths by scheduling time to do two of the discovery activities we've discussed. Write down the event, date, time, and leave room to record what you've learned after.

Event

_____

_____

Time

_____

_____

Date

_____

_____

Reflection

_____

_____

_____

_____

Developing Your Skills

Don't forget that college provides opportunities for you to home in your skills inside and outside of the classroom. The skills you're learning in class—like critical thinking and how to communicate and write clearly—can complement the skills you learn in activities you do outside of school like volunteering, clubs, and internships. Even if you're doing something for fun, you're bound to be developing and showcasing something that will benefit you in the future!

Hard Skills

Hard skills are learned skills that can be defined, evaluated, and measured, and focus on specific knowledge necessary to perform a job. Some examples of hard skills include UX design, video production, and proposal writing. College is here to help you develop these skills. You're learning new concepts and techniques in a degree or certificate program that shows your mastery in a discipline. On the other side of the spectrum are soft skills.

The Hard Question

What are some of your biggest hard skill strengths?

1. _____

2. _____

3. _____

Soft Skills

Soft skills are the attributes you can contribute that are not technical, like problem solving, adaptability, and resiliency. These are the traits that you don't earn a degree in, but you build over time through experiences and overcoming challenges. Soft skills are usually harder to teach in a position, so if you're particularly strong on soft skills, it's smart to frame it as something that would be extremely beneficial to an employer. As a college student, especially if your experience is a bit limited, soft skills can be your ticket to boosting your chances of landing an internship or job.

Career

Soft Skills, Strong Resume

What are some of your biggest soft skill strengths?

1. _____

2. _____

3. _____

Career Center Services

Career centers have resources for you to use throughout your college career (and sometimes after!). Applying for a part-time job or internship? Hoping to get into a competitive PhD program or land your first full-time job? They can help. Each school has their own services, but here are some of the most common and how you can get a leg up on the competition.

Resume Services

A college resume can be made up of awards and recognitions, activities, and experiences that showcase your talents and skills. College career or writing centers will help you get started, and even guide you in creating an online professional presence. You will need to update your resume often as you progress through college. While it may seem intimidating and time consuming, it's a lot easier to revisit this living document after the end of every term rather than once a year and trying to remember everything you've done.

If you're working in college at a job that's unrelated to your career goals, which is totally normal and financially savvy by the way, it's still a part of your resume and you can even write your skills in a way that are applicable to a career, even if it's in a different field. Example: You're majoring in business and you're aiming for a job in international relations. You currently work at a coffee shop. Which resume description sounds more impressive?

Resume 1:

Job experience **The Daily Brew**

Lead barista serving customers various drinks, opening and closing the store, responsible for training new baristas.

Resume 2:
Job experience

The Daily Brew

- One of the first college students to earn lead barista.

- Utilized bilingual skills to communicate with customers.

- Organized shifts and led team meetings.

- Increased store sales and customer base by organizing store events and promotions.

- Trained and led new employees to meet company-wide goals and customer service standards.

With a simple restructure, your resume can stand out regardless of your experience. Your student resume can have a few different experiences, including things like volunteering, student clubs, campus jobs, internships, research, and even your academic standing. As you progress and ultimately graduate, your resume will begin to look a bit more fluid, but it's helpful to know that regardless of where you are, you can get help with shining it up a bit.

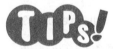

Here are some things to keep in mind while updating your resume.

- Write a clear objective statement. This can be a few sentences that help the reader know your larger goals, like the career path you're aiming for, or your areas of study.

- Note your strengths, experiences, and skill sets.

- Demonstrate growth over the years.

- Put your education, where you're studying and the expected date of graduation, plus any relevant coursework.

- Focus on your impact within the activity or job you've held.

- Start sentences with strong action verbs.

- Add any professional organizations that you belong to.

- If you have a professional profile on a platform like LinkedIn or Handshake, make sure to keep those "online resumes" up to date.

- Always proofread your final drafts.

- When in doubt, get advice from a professional at the career center.

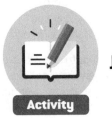

Activity

Job Posting

Read the following job posting and tailor one section of your resume (previous work experience, volunteer work, clubs & activities, etc.) to the job. Write three bullet points for the section you choose.

Research Position—Full Time; Over Summer

Students will have an opportunity to complete an 8-week summer field work joining an active research team completing the following tasks; data science for psychology department, communicating and organizing focus groups for clinical trials, working closely with professors and graduate students.

- _____

- _____

- _____

Job Search Support

Work experience is a great way to get hands-on experience in an industry while simultaneously developing new skills and applying what you've learned in school. But where do you start? Your career center has lots of tools to help you locate available opportunities and help you work your way through the application processes.

Jobs can take many forms: internships, part-time work, full-time jobs, and even volunteer work. Depending on your wants and needs, your advisors might recommend certain paths. For example, you might want to study abroad and complete an internship while in college, so your career advisor helps you coordinate with the study abroad office to identify and enroll in a for-credit summer internship abroad. Alternatively, volunteering at the school clinic or local hospital is a great way to show med schools that you're committed to learning all you can and helping your community. There are so many types of work available; the key is doing the research to find the perfect fit. Our biggest tip? Don't limit yourself! Here's how:

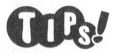

■ Ask about opportunities with a set time frame (i.e., January term internships, semester-long volunteer work, summer jobs, etc.) so you can plan for the additional commitment.

■ Find out what's available through your college, such as for-credit or on-campus internships, university exchanges, community partnerships, etc.

■ Think about where you spend your summers and school year and ask a career counselor to help you find opportunities in those communities.

■ If a work opportunity is unpaid or has related expenses, seek out scholarships or grants to help make up the costs. Your career center can direct you to school-sponsored and outside help.

Career

The work you put into securing volunteer work, internships, and part-time jobs is worth it. In the end, assuming you put in your best effort, you'll usually walk away with a fantastic learning experience and a new connection that could provide you a reference or let you know of a full-time opportunity one day.

Interview Preparation

Career counselors can help you practice for interviews. Mock interviews are often available and easy to schedule. You can literally go through the entire process, from dressing up for the interview and walking in all the way to introducing yourself and answering questions. Some colleges will also tailor career preparation towards your major. Business majors might have an opportunity to practice a dinner out with a potential client or employer, for example. Maybe you have an interview that is happening online rather in person. The feeling on camera could be more awkward than in person. Practicing logging on, speaking through a camera, and still commanding a strong practice. These are all tools to help you feel confident for when it is time to interview.

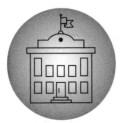

COLLEGE SPOTLIGHT

High Point University is all about providing realistic situations to help students feel prepared for applying, pitching themselves for a potential job, and interviewing. At the on-campus fine dining restaurant called 1924 Prime, students will make a reservation, dress professionally, leave their phones off during the meal, and practice etiquette in what could potentially be a lunch or dinner interview. Beyond the restaurant, one of the student cafes literally has a fake airplane with seats, and windows for students to use and feel comfortable networking and making small talk with others. You never know who you're sitting next to in life, and by practicing your elevator pitches, or an informal interview, and networking skills with your peers can help you feel equipped for the real thing.

Networking Resources

When you have the benefit of a larger university, networking can be a game changer. Networking widens your professional and social contacts by getting to know others and exchanging ideas and information. It can simply be an introduction and a follow-up email that might later down the line turn into a prospective internship referral or a mentor.

Go to all the speaker series and speaker sessions your school offers, meet alumni when you can to network with them, and explore the city where you live. Grades are important but not the end all be all, so expand your network and enjoy!

—Carli, University of California, Berkeley

Alumni Networks

Your university has an alumni network. These are individuals who have graduated from the university and are now working professionals. Let's say your university is out of state from your hometown, and your goal after graduation is to land a position back home. You might check out alumni in related professions based out of your local area and reach out to them for a coffee over summer break. Faculty and peers can also be a part of your network. The student sitting next to you in creative writing might one day be a business partner. The professor teaching intro to engineering might write you a recommendation letter for your first job.

Career

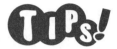

Here's a few tips to guide you while networking:

- Introduce yourself and what you're studying, or what year you are.

- When you meet someone new, repeat their name back to remember it better. Example: *Hi, I'm Michael. Hi Michael, it's nice to meet you!*

- Find a common ground with the person you're speaking with. Are you both studying the same subject? Are they also passionate about a certain field or subject?

- Instead of outright asking about someone's professional experience, ask about their interests, why they went into the field they did, what they value about their work, etc. By digging deeper, you're creating more meaningful conversations rather than a resume list.

- Once you've connected with someone, thank them for the conversation and ask for a business card or an email.

- Follow up with the person! The last thing you want to do is email someone that you haven't talked to in a while and right away ask for a reference or a job opportunity. A simple email saying hello, sharing your most recent experiences, and asking about their work can build a stronger relationship.

- If you find yourself feeling really nervous, or anxious, remind yourself this isn't an interview. All you're doing is getting to know new people. There is nothing to lose and only good to gain, even if it's simply a small conversation.

- Ensure your online presence is up to date and reflective of what you want people to see. Check your social media accounts. If they're public, are you comfortable if a future employer sees what's posted?

REFLECTION

Using your current or intended major, write down a list of possible careers based on your research, conversations, and findings. Explain how you feel about these opportunities.

_____

_____

_____

_____

_____

Review your resume and identify one way to strengthen it. Be specific (learn a specific skill, join a professional club or an organization within your field, take on a leadership role, etc.) and write out your plan to achieve your goal.

_____

_____

_____

_____

_____

Career

CHAPTER 11

Finances

Whether you receive financial support from family and friends, grants and scholarships, or are taking on debt and part-time work to fund your college years, this chapter will leave you feeling more confident about your expenses. While college can be considered as an investment, feeling the financial burden from student loans and managing day-to-day expenses can make for a mentally exhausting few years. This chapter will dissect your overall personal and school-related expenses and narrow in on a few money-saving and strategizing tips, as well as making sure you are aware of resources in case you find yourself in a financial emergency or hardship.

Your friends invite you on a weekend ski trip, and you couldn't be more excited for a real break. The mountains are about an hour away, and you love skiing, but don't have all of your gear. As you start adding up the rental fees, cost of food, transportation, and housing, you start feeling like it might be a little steep, and we're not talking about the mountain. You've been saving money for a while now, but how do you decide if this is worth tapping into those funds when you have other expenses to worry about?

You're coming up at the end of your first year. You're ecstatic that you've made it through successfully, but are a bit panicked as to how to afford next year's tuition. You had some scholarships from high school that covered a few costs, but they won't roll over, and you still have a gap between what the college has offered you financially. You begin to feel a bit disheartened and don't want to think about the prospect of transferring, especially now that you finally feel a bit more at home. What options do you even have? It's not like money grows on trees.

Introduction

While you can expect horror stories about walking into class late or trying to make plans for the weekend to come up in your conversations with friends, odds are the topic of finances is rarely included in those chats. To be fair, conversation starters that begin with "So, how are you handling your student loans?" aren't necessarily captivating, but if students *did* share their fears, it might feel better to know that it's not uncommon.

Seventy percent of college students worry about having enough money to pay for school.

Everything from the cost of tuition and housing to textbook fees and money for meals can snowball into one giant financial stressor, especially when you add on extra costs like social activities and traveling back home.

It might feel taboo to talk about money, but it can also be frustrating trying to learn how to manage your expenses and build a budget when you have no experience or guidance, and what's on the Internet feels out of touch. Sure, you can get a coffee machine and save on buying lattes; that's simple enough. But that doesn't solve the massive burden of student loans, make you feel more confident handling larger financial decisions, or help you get your day-to-day expenses under control. Ultimately, when you feel pressured financially, it's hard to focus on schoolwork and life.

Finances

This chapter will help reiterate that you are not alone. *A lot* of students have added financial strain due to factors like drastic income changes, unexpected costs, and emergencies. You'll learn how to get a hold of your expenses, so that you can build a budget that works for you and helps you manage your money. In this chapter, you'll also get tips and exercises for identifying resources to turn to if financial challenges come your way. This is your opportunity to get familiar and comfortable with your finances, regardless of where you attend and how much money you currently have.

Planning

Just like you're planning for a future career by pursuing a particular academic track, you should also use this time to build a financial plan. Now that you have a better understanding of your current expenses, it'll be a lot easier to build out a budget and create a plan for both short-term and long-term financial goals. This can be as big as picking a student loan repayment plan or building an emergency fund, or something smaller if you're just starting out, like putting the utilities in your name so you can build credit. As you figure all of these things out, it's also good to remind yourself that you're still learning. You will make mistakes, but don't be too hard on yourself because part of learning is trying something and getting it wrong. You can take your mess-ups and money blinders and turn them around so you feel better about your situation.

Building a Budget

A budget is a tool you can use to track your expenses and income and helps you live within your means. You're already part way to building out a budget from estimating your expenses. The next step is to put it into action. Pick a few weeks or a few months and track every transaction to see if your estimations aligned with your actual spending habits. This way, you'll be able to notice trends in your finances, like months where you spend more on transportation or less on food. By tracking your actual habits with money, you'll know how to adjust your allocations and where you can cut down if need be. Use these tips to help you get started.

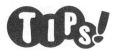

■ Mark deadlines for things like completing the FAFSA, applying for scholarships, or when your bills are due. Also mark days you can expect a paycheck.

■ Categorize your expenses in a way that makes sense to you so it's easier to track.

■ Keep an organized spreadsheet or download an app to store your monthly history and keep you within budget as the month progresses.

■ Didn't break even? Look to see if you can reallocate funds for certain areas or cut other expenses entirely.

Handling Debt

You may be carrying various types of debt: student loans, medical debt, or credit card debt. Each of these can be stressful in their own ways but learning about the terms of your repayments can help you figure out a strategic plan. You might see finance articles talk about "good debt" and "bad debt," and while it may be a bit of a simplification (too much debt of any kind can be troublesome!), essentially it divides your debt into low-interest debt that can help increase your income and reach your goals, like student debt, and expensive debts that make your finances worse, like credit card debt. Of course, it would be great if you had no debt, but sometimes that just is not possible! If you find yourself overwhelmed by your debt, reach out to your providers to talk about special repayment plans or look for financial literacy classes at your school or in your community. The sooner you seek assistance, the sooner you'll be able to be back on track.

Saving

If you can start putting some money into savings when you're in school, it'll help you in the long run. Whether you're building an emergency fund, saving for a post-graduation move, or just want to buy a go-to interview outfit, use these tips to help you get started.

Finances

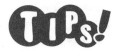

- Put a little money away each month, whether that's $50 or $5. Each bit adds up!

- Keep your savings in a separate account that you won't touch until it's time to cash in.

- Hold your funds in an account that builds interest so it can grow faster.

- Research what type of savings tools—like a high yield savings account, CD, stocks, Roth IRA, etc.—best fits your goals.

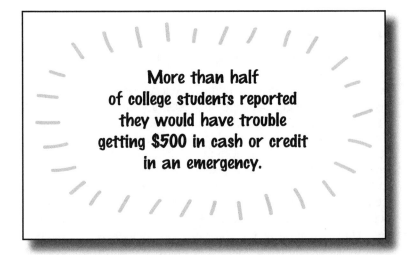

More than half
of college students reported
they would have trouble
getting $500 in cash or credit
in an emergency.

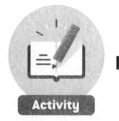

Activity

Budget Worksheet

Fill in the empty spaces or take the worksheet and create your own.

Income	
	$
	$
	$
Total Income =	$
Expense	
Tuition and Fees	$
Housing	$
Meals	$
Textbooks	$
Transportation and Travel	$
Medical	$
Activities	$
Fun Money	$
Total Expense =	$
Total Income – Total Expense = Amount Leftover	$

Looking at your amount leftover, how are you going to use that money or reallocate your funds to hit even?

_____

_____

_____

Managing Expenses

As you prepare for college, you might have spent some time looking for scholarships and completing financial aid forms, but once you're in, how often do you pause and check in on your financial situation? Understanding your current financial health is an important part of managing your money in college, as it allows you to maximize your resources. The best place to begin this process is by taking an honest look at your expenses. By reviewing all of the money you are spending, both small and large sums, you'll be able to see where your wallet is fixed and where you can strategize to save.

School-Related Expenses

According to our College Hopes & Worries survey, the cost of attendance is the biggest concern for prospective college students, so it's no surprise that the stress of school-related expenses might weigh heavily on your mind during your college years. These expenses include books, room and board, tuition, transportation, lab fees, add/drop fees, student fees, and...why are there so many fees?! Although addressing all school-related expenses can be overwhelming or even upsetting, it'll not only help you come up with a plan now, but better prepare you both financially and emotionally for handling any debt after you graduate. Here are some types of school-related expenses to help get you familiar with some college costs.

Tuition and Fees

It's worth checking your tuition and fees each year to see if there are expenses you don't need to pay or that might have some flexibility. Start by logging onto your online portal or getting a copy of your financial aid package to review each cost and check for optional or repetitive fees. For example, health insurance is often included in your total cost of attendance. It might be an automatic line item with a hefty bill so that you're covered health wise, but if you're under your parents' insurance, you might not have to pay for the university's insurance. You'd essentially be paying double for a service you already have. Another optional fee you can reevaluate is your room and board plan. Are you living in the most expensive housing option and meal plan? Maybe you eat out or cook more at home than you thought, or maybe you like the idea of living in non-campus housing and find out it's less expensive. Either way, looking at these flexible accommodation fees can allow you to save money based on your living preferences.

Textbooks

Books and supplies can cost upward of a thousand dollars, but you can often save hundreds by getting creative with resources available to you. Check out these tips for how to save on your textbooks.

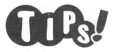

- Ask your professors if the current edition is mandatory for the class, or if you can use a previous edition, which is usually less expensive.

- Buy used, discounted textbooks online or at your campus bookstore. (Alternatively, see if there's a job opening at the bookstore, as that generally comes not only with a paycheck but a discount.)

- Compare prices at different stores before you buy and find out if any of them offer price matching.

- Share books with peers in the same class.

- Purchase online editions rather than the hard copy.

- Rent your textbooks for the semester.

- Look for student book swap groups online, on social media, etc.

- Check the library to see if current copies of textbooks are available to check out.

Finances

Personal Expenses

Personal expenses can include a variety of costs including transportation and travel, medical, activities, and fun money. Typically, you have more flexibility with your personal expenses because they are set by you and not your institution. As you evaluate these costs, keep in mind that you should not only consider what's important and financially doable, but how it impacts your overall happiness. Know your priorities and adjust your personal expenses to match. Let's look at some of the personal expense categories to get you started.

Transportation and Travel

These expenses will fluctuate depending on your living situation and other factors. If you live within walking distance to everything on campus, you're going to be paying less for transportation during the school week. Similarly, you can weigh the convenience of having a car on campus with the costs of a parking pass, insurance, and gas. You might find that you'd be happy using public transportation or realize that you'd spend too much money on rideshare services getting home from the store, activities, or day trips. Each person's cost benefit analysis will look different, so focus on what fits your needs best.

If you plan to go home during the academic year, it's also important to factor in travel expenses. Keep an eye out for carpooling options for people traveling in the same direction or to the same city and set a tracker on flights to make sure you can purchase one when the rates are low.

Medical

Medical expenses can be hard to predict. If you're currently taking medications, it's important to make sure you factor this cost into your budget. For your safety, do not stop taking your medication without consulting your doctor first; but if you find that your medicine is more expensive than you can afford, talk to your doctor about generic equivalents or go online for discount coupons to help reduce costs.

We can't talk about medical expenses without touching on health insurance. Health insurance is complicated for everyone. Assess your current health insurance plan—Are you still on your parents' insurance? Do you need to get your own?—and see what you're working with. There are a lot of technical terms that can sound intimidating, which makes it all the more tempting to just ignore them. Don't! Learn about your coverage so you aren't hit with medical bills that you weren't anticipating. All insurance companies have customer service lines where you can ask for clarification about your benefits, coverage, costs, and more.

Here are some of the fundamental terms you should look out for and why they're important in saving you money.

- **In-Network:** An in-network healthcare provider has a contract with your health insurance plan to provide health-care services to its plan members at a pre-negotiated rate. If you can, try to stay in-network for providers, pharmacies, and hospitals so that you can keep your medical care costs down.

- **Deductible:** This is a fixed amount of money that you must pay towards applicable medical expenses in a coverage period before your insurance will cover the costs. For example, if your deductible is $750, you must pay $750 before your insurance kicks in. If you can set aside a medical emergency fund to cover your deductible, you will feel more confident in your ability to cover this medical expense.

- **Co-Insurance:** This is the percentage of costs of a covered healthcare service you pay after you've paid your deductible. For example, if you've paid the $750 deductible above, and you now have a $100 office visit and a coinsurance of 20%, your total cost would be $20. It's important to evaluate your insurance every year to know what your cost-sharing responsibilities are prior to being hit with an unexpected bill.

Finances

- **Copay:** This is a flat rate you pay for a service. For example, a specialty service like a visit to the dermatologist might cost you $30. While this is a fixed rate, sometimes you can find discounts that make something less expensive than your copay. Always do your research!

- **Preventative Service:** While not a complicated term, this one is important to know. All insurance plans must cover certain preventative services, such as specific injections and wellness exams, assuming they are in-network. Know your healthcare rights and reach out to your insurance company if you believe you have been billed unfairly or incorrectly.

Activities

You might join a club or a team that has fees for things like travel expenses, gear, or various events that go on throughout the semester. When you're looking to join a club or activity, make sure to learn about these expenses beforehand and ask if they change every semester or year. If you want to participate but cannot afford the full amount, check to see if you can go on a payment plan or if there's any financial help available for those facing financial hardship.

Fun Money

You can think of fun money as money spent on things you want, but don't need. This can include vacations, subscription services, eating out, and more. It's important to allow yourself some fun money because even though it's an expense, by treating yourself to something you enjoy, you're less likely to go overboard from being too restrictive and unrealistic. Just make sure your fun budget isn't putting you into substantial debt or causing you to neglect necessities.

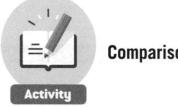

Comparison Shopping

Activity

Your old laptop finally died on you, and it's time to invest in a new one. This is one of your first big expenses, so you want to a do a bit of research before buying. Follow the steps to help you compare your purchase options. Use your current spending habits as a guide for your purchasing power.

Think of factors that are important to you when considering which laptop to purchase. List and rank your top five, with position one being the highest.

Important Factor Brainstorming	Top Five Factors	Ranking (1–5)

Finances

Next, insert your top factors into the table below. Identify three vendors and score them (up to 10 points for each factor) on how well they satisfy the factors you deemed most important in your purchase.

Factor	Vendor 1	Vendor 2	Vendor 3
	Total Points:	Total Points:	Total Points:

Based on this exercise, which vendor are you going to go with and why?

_____

_____

_____

_____

How does weighing your wants and needs impact your expenses?

_____

_____

_____

_____

Financial Hardship and Emergencies

If you find yourself in a really tough spot, like trouble with consistent housing, not enough money to purchase food, etc., reach out to your university for support. Speak with an advisor or a counselor who can refer you to free support services on campus that will help in an emergency or guide you out of a crisis. Your university is a resource, so while you're paying to be there, get the most out of all that's available to you. That includes financial aid experts that will help you understand loans, strategize your finances, and help you when in need.

Finding More Money

As you go throughout each term, opportunities to earn money and save money can present themselves, so be vigilant about seeking them out along the way. Here are some places you can look to help get you going.

FAFSA

Each year, you'll want to complete the Free Application for Federal Student Aid (FAFSA) and other forms your university requires so that you can be considered for financial aid. This form will notify your school of your family's income, and it can open up doors for more financial support if your family is facing new economic hardships or a change in income. Types of tuition support can fluctuate depending on things like financial need so it's important to apply each year and work with your financial aid office if circumstances change.

Grants and Scholarships

Grants and scholarships are two things that can be awarded in your financial aid package, but you should also check for these throughout each term. Check with your academic department for competitions and scholarship opportunities within your area of

Finances

expertise, and also stop by the financial aid office for a reputable resource on researching scholarships locally and nationally. You never know what you'll receive so don't be afraid to ask and apply.

Federal Work-Study

Federal work-study is awarded to students as part of their financial aid package through the department of education. If you qualify, there's a few perks to the job and things to consider:

- You can get various jobs on campus working for departments or the school, and even off campus opportunities with an affiliated nonprofit organization or department.

- You still need to apply and interview for jobs in most cases.

- The earnings you make through work study do not count against you on your next FAFSA, which means you won't be deducted for making more income.

- Your employer will work with your class schedule and you'll have a limited number of hours.

- There can be limited funding and less jobs available, so if you're finding it's not matching up, you can still search for a job otherwise.

Academics

Graduating on time (and sometimes early!), is a great way to save money on extra years of college expenses. Did you know that according to the most recent data, over 60% of students will complete their bachelor's degree in six years? That adds a big tuition bill leaving you with potentially taking on more loans, or investing in more than you initially planned. Here's a few tips to keep you on track.

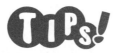

- Meet regularly with an academic advisor to stay on track of coursework and see if there are any classes you can skip due to proficiency or take a course that will count both for major coursework and to fulfill a requirement.

- Check to see if you can take a community college class that is transferable. You could take one class, for example, over the summer when you're back home at a lower rate at your local community college, knocking out some credits for less.

- Find out if your school charges a flat rate tuition for a range of credits and try to take as many credits as you can manage. For example, if your school charges $10,000 for 12-18 credits, try to take on an extra class to get you closer to 18 credits.

Work

Whether you're making fancy lattes or tutoring, finding work is a way a lot of students support themselves and pocket some extra cash. There's a few different types of work you can apply for and while getting a job helps manage costs, it's important to prioritize academics and manage your time so you can still get some sleep, study, and stay sane with a social life.

Part-Time

Working part-time means that you're not allowed to work more than 35 hours per week. You can work any number of hours below 35 as deemed appropriate by your employer, but most shifts tend to a few hours at a time. Part-time jobs are usually plentiful both on-campus and in the surrounding community. The key with part-time work is being able to find a position where you can balance your school commitments with your work commitments. Be on top of your schedule and communicate to your boss when you need to be scheduled for fewer hours long in advance.

Finances

Freelance

Freelance work allows you to take on work on a project-to-project basis, or on your own time. If you're crafty, this might look like putting together embroidery kits to sell on Etsy. Alternatively, if you're a great writer, this could be writing articles or content for company or organizational websites. Though it can be hard to get started, freelancing gives you a lot of control over the time you commit to work.

Occasional

Maybe any kind of long-term commitment to a job stresses you out. That's totally fine! There are plenty of one-off jobs or opportunities that can help you earn some cash fast. You can find ads for people in need of childcare or moving assistance, or even paid research studies that you can participate in as a subject. Keep your eye on the school classifieds and jump at an opportunity if it interests you.

Remember not to bite off more than you can chew...
Make a weekly/monthly schedule and know when to work
fewer hours in order to make sure you don't burn out.
Also, something that I found really helpful is to schedule
2–3 hours a week of "me time"... This will help you a lot with
stress management and self-awareness.

—Mary, University of Massachusetts, Amherst

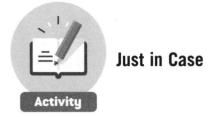

Activity

Just in Case

Write strategies and list where you can go for the following in case you're struggling to make ends meet. It's OK if you don't fully know the answer yet, but it's important to think ahead so you're prepared!

1. Name at least one person you can turn to for financial guidance and help:

   _____

   _____

2. If you are having trouble affording expenses at the start of a term (like getting books, supplies, trouble paying travel costs back to campus), what are some strategies you can take?

   _____

   _____

3. Need help with housing:

   _____

   _____

4. If an emergency happens and you need money fast:

   _____

   _____

Finances

5. Help completing financial aid forms (like FAFSA and others) that are quite confusing:

_____

_____

6. Food:

_____

_____

7. Medical Care:

_____

_____

8. Help building a savings account and don't know where to invest:

_____

_____

REFLECTION

How comfortable and familiar are you with your monthly expenses? What is one area in which you can reduce your spending?

_____

_____

_____

_____

List three long- or short-term financial goals (i.e. build an emergency fund, pay off credit card debt, etc.). Be specific! What is one step you can take to reach these goals?

_____

_____

_____

_____

How do you feel about working while in school? List the pros and cons of taking on a job.

_____

_____

_____

_____

Finances

How comfortable are you financially? Write out your three biggest fears when it comes to financial insecurity and the steps you can take to address them.

_____

_____

_____

_____

About the Author

Casey Rowley Barneson holds a Master's degree in Educational Counseling and is currently the college counselor at Beverly Hills High School and an adjunct professor with the University of La Verne. For over ten years, she has worked within the education system and directly with families to navigate the college admission process, from preparation and planning to applying and gaining admission. She has also participated on college advisory boards and served on the board of a non-profit scholars program to help provide access to students with limited college counseling. Additionally, she is an active member and presenter for the National Association for College Admission Counseling and Western Association for College Admission Counseling, which allows her to travel to colleges and universities worldwide as she follows her passion to help students discover their best-fit colleges. She maintains an active blog at www.collegecounselorrowley.com.